£13 80p NETT

150 N

Received R. T. Department Date

Students Library   121

D1350043

Gallium-67 Imaging

Wiley Series in Diagnostic and Therapeutic Radiology

Luther W. Brady, M.D., Editor
*Professor and Chairman, Department of Therapeutic Radiology
and Nuclear Medicine, Hahnemann Medical College and
Hospital, Philadelphia, Pennsylvania*

Gallium-67 Imaging

Edited by

Paul B. Hoffer, M.D.

Director of Nuclear Medicine
Professor of Diagnostic Radiology
Yale University School of Medicine
New Haven, Connecticut

Carlos Bekerman, M.D.

Assistant Professor of Radiology
and Medicine
University of Chicago–
Pritzker School of Medicine
Chicago, Illinois

Robert E. Henkin, M.D.

Director of Nuclear Medicine
Assistant Professor of Radiology
Foster G. McGaw Hospital
Loyola University Medical Center
Maywood, Illinois

A WILEY MEDICAL PUBLICATION
JOHN WILEY & SONS
New York • Chichester • Brisbane • Toronto

Copyright © 1978 by John Wiley & Sons, Inc.

All rights reserved. Published simultaneously in Canada.

No part of this book may be reproduced by any means, nor transmitted, nor translated into a machine language without the written permission of the publisher.

Library of Congress Cataloging in Publication Data:

Gallium-67 Imaging.

    (Wiley series in diagnostic and therapeutic radiology.)
    Includes bibliographical references and index.
    1. Cancer—Diagnosis. 2. Inflammation—Diagnosis.
3. Radioisotope scanning. 4. Gallium—Isotopes.
I. Hoffer, Paul B. II. Bekerman, Carlos.
III. Henkin, Robert E.
RC270.G34   616.07'575   77-13125
ISBN 0-471-02601-8

Printed in the United States of America

10 9 8 7 6 5 4 3 2 1

Contributors

Carlos Bekerman, M.D., Clinical Staff, Division of Nuclear Medicine, Michael Reese Hospital and Medical Center; Assistant Professor of Radiology and Medicine, University of Chicago-Pritzker School of Medicine, Chicago, Illinois 60616

Robert J. Churchill, M.D., Assistant Clinical Professor of Radiology, Foster G. McGaw Hospital, Loyola University Medical Center, Maywood, Illinois 60153

Ernest W. Fordham, M.D., Professor of Nuclear Medicine and Radiology, Rush Medical College; Chairman, Department of Nuclear Medicine, Rush-Presbyterian–St. Luke's Medical Center, Chicago, Illinois 60612

Robert E. Henkin, M.D., Director of Nuclear Medicine, Assistant Professor of Radiology, Foster G. McGaw Hospital, Loyola University Medical Center, Maywood, Illinois 60153

Paul B. Hoffer, M.D., Professor of Diagnostic Radiology, Director, Section of Nuclear Medicine, Yale University School of Medicine, New Haven, Connecticut 06510

Steven M. Larson, M.D., Assistant Chief of Nuclear Medicine, Veterans Administration Hospital; Associate Professor of Medicine, Laboratory Medicine and Radiology, University of Washington, Seattle, Washington 98102

Steven M. Pinsky, M.D., Director, Division of Nuclear Medicine, Michael Reese Hospital and Medical Center; Associate Professor of Radiology and Medicine, University of Chicago–Pritzker School of Medicine, Chicago, Illinois 60616

Carlos J. Reynes, M.D., Director of Ultrasound and Whole Body Computed Tomography, Associate Professor of Radiology, Foster G. McGaw Hospital, Loyola University Medical Center, Maywood, Illinois 60153

Robert E. Slayton, M.D., Associate Professor of Medicine, Rush Medical College, Department of Nuclear Medicine, Rush-Presbyterian–St. Luke's Medical Center, Chicago, Illinois 60612

David A. Turner, M.D., Associate Professor of Nuclear Medicine and Radiology, Rush Medical College; Department of Nuclear Medicine, Rush-Presbyterian–St. Luke's Medical Center, Chicago, Illinois 60612

Series Preface

The past five years have produced an explosion in the knowledge, techniques, and clinical application of radiology in all of its specialties. New techniques in diagnostic radiology have contributed to a quality of medical care for the patient unparalleled in the United States. Among these techniques are the development and applications in ultrasound, the development and implementation of computed tomography, and many exploratory studies using holographic techniques. The advances in nuclear medicine have allowed for a wider diversity of application of these techniques in clinical medicine and have involved not only major new developments in instrumentation, but also development of newer radiopharmaceuticals.

Advances in radiation therapy have significantly improved the cure rates for cancer. Radiation techniques in the treatment of cancer are now utilized in more than 50% of the patients with the established diagnosis of cancer.

It is the purpose of this series of monographs to bring together the various aspects of radiology and all its specialties so that the physician by continuance of his education and rigid self-discipline may maintain high standards of professional knowledge.

LUTHER W. BRADY, M.D.

Preface

The story of gallium-67 imaging is an interesting example of the role of seren-dipity in the progress of medicine. When Edwards and Hayes initiated their studies of gallium-67, they were primarily interested in its use as a bone-scanning agent (1). Thus, if the development of the ^{99m}Tc-labeled phosphate compounds occurred only a few years earlier (2), the original clinical studies of gallium-67 might never have been undertaken. While Edwards and Hayes must have been disappointed in the mediocre bone-localizing characteristics of their carrier-free gallium-67, they were quick to recognize the significance of the unexpected deposition of the radionuclide in tumor.

As gallium-67 began to be used clinically for tumor imaging, numerous inves-tigators noticed that it not only localized in malignant tissue but in inflammatory lesions as well. It remained, however, for Lavender (3) and Littenberg (4) and their associates to exploit these "false positives" into an entirely new field of gallium imaging.

In spite of the fact that much of the basic clinical investigative work has been accomplished, it is still difficult for even the most dedicated practitioner to keep track of the expanding body of information on gallium imaging. New applica-tions have been introduced, some older applications have not stood the test of time, new mechanisms of localization have been proposed, and even the deter-mination of the energy of the major photon emissions has been in a state of flux. Changes in techniques have been introduced which have significant conse-quences on scan interpretation. The same pattern of distribution which is nor-mal for the 24-hour image may be distinctly abnormal for the 72-hour image. Moreover, important information about gallium may appear in a variety of journals, many of which are not frequently read by physicians who practice nuclear medicine.

Therefore, the purpose of this book is to bring together in one concise volume the state of the art in the clinical use of gallium. While it will not be the last word on gallium, we hope it does serve as convenient primer and reference source.

PAUL B. HOFFER, M.D.
CARLOS BEKERMAN, M.D.
ROBERT E. HENKIN, M.D.

REFERENCES

1. Subramanian G, McAfee JG: A new complex of ^{99m}Tc for skeletal imaging. *Radiology* 98:192, 1971.
2. Edwards CL and Hayes RL: Tumor scanning with gallium citrate. *J Nucl Med* 10:103, 1969.
3. Lavender JP, Barker JR, and Chaudhri MA: Gallium-67 citrate scanning in neoplastic and inflammatory lesions. *Br. J Radiol* 44:361, 1971.
4. Littenberg RL, Taketa RM, Alazraki NP et al: Gallium-67 for the localization of septic lesions. *Ann Int Med* 79:403, 1973.

Acknowledgments

While we, the editors, assume responsibility for the contents of this volume, it is both our duty and our privilege to acknowledge the people who helped us. One person in particular, Mrs. Elizabeth White, has spent a great amount of time and effort on this project. In addition to her usual task of supervising a busy office, she has also prepared much of the original manuscript; she organized, proofread, edited, coordinated, and retyped the contributed chapters, and then put the entire work in final form for publication. The book could not have been put together without her.

We are also grateful to Dr. Luther Brady, who originally proposed that this book be written and who facilitated its publication. Drs. James L. Quinn III and Alexander Gottschalk were instrumental in establishing the refresher course from which the format of the book evolved. Finally, we are indebted to John deCarville, Kathy Nelson, Maura Fitzgerald and their staff at John Wiley & Sons for their kind treatment of the editors and the text.

PAUL B. HOFFER
CARLOS BEKERMAN
ROBERT E. HENKIN

Contents

Gallium-67 Imaging

Part 1
Fundamentals

1
Mechanisms of Localization

Paul B. Hoffer, M.D.

Professor of Diagnostic Radiology
Director, Section of Nuclear Medicine
Yale University School of Medicine
New Haven, Connecticut

Many fundamental aspects of gallium-67 (^{67}Ga) transport and localization are unknown. When ^{67}Ga citrate is injected intravenously, much of the dose binds loosely to plasma protein, while some remains in soluble citrate configuration (1–3). Gallium-67 is bound primarily to transferrin and other α- and β-serum globulins. The extent of binding is dependent on numerous factors. Increase in both citrate content (above 6.6 μmol of citrate per 10 ml of serum) and carrier gallium content decreases the extent of plasma protein binding (1). Interestingly, increases in carrier gallium and citrate content have also been found to decrease localization of gallium in tumors. Iron also competes with gallium for binding sites on transferrin. Excess iron blocks ^{67}Ga binding to transferrin. If serum transferrin is saturated with iron at the time of ^{67}Ga citrate injection, tumor uptake of the radionuclide is inhibited. Paradoxically, administration of iron 24 hours after administration of ^{67}Ga citrate actually enhances tumor to background ratios (4). When ^{67}Ga citrate is administered to patients with saturated transferrin-binding sites, less localization in liver, greater renal activity, and more rapid clearance (Figure 1) occur. Scandium, administered coincidentally with ^{67}Ga citrate, also blocks protein binding of the radionuclide. However, in this case, tumor to background ratios are enhanced. Unfortunately, the doses of scandium required to enhance tumor to background ratios also cause hemolysis of human erythrocytes; therefore, this method of enhancing ^{67}Ga imaging is not clinically useful (5–7).

Approximately 15–25% of ^{67}Ga is excreted by the kidneys within the first 24 hours after intravenous injection. Clearance of radioactivity from the body after the first 24 hours is usually slow. The remaining ^{67}Ga is distributed in the plasma and body tissues and retained for several weeks; its biologic half-life is approximately 25 days (8,9). After 24 hours, the major route of excretion is the colon.

Swartzendruber et al. (10), by use of ultracentrifugation, originally determined that the intracellular localization of ^{67}Ga occurred in lysosomes or lysosome-like granules of the cell. Aulbert and associates (11) confirmed

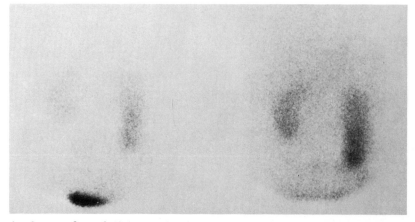

Figure 1.   Scan performed 48 hours after ^{67}Ga injection in patient with hemochromatosis. No hepatic, splenic, or bone activity is observed. Only kidney and some bowel activity are detectable. This abnormal pattern of ^{67}Ga localization in patients with hemochromatosis supports the concept that ^{67}Ga acts in certain respects as an iron analog.

lysosomal localization of ^{67}Ga in the liver. Subsequent ultracentrifugation studies (12) demonstrated that normal tissues, such as the liver, localized ^{67}Ga in the lysosomal fraction. Animal hepatomas and lymphosarcomas, however, localized ^{67}Ga not only in lysosomes but also in smaller cellular particles that are associated with the endoplasmic reticulum and in small, electron-dense, single-membrane granules. Ito and colleagues (13) showed a somewhat different pattern of intracellular localization. They found significant quantities of ^{67}Ga in soluble fractions and bound to nuclear, mitochondrial, and microsomal cell components. They also demonstrated preferential localization in viable, as compared to nonviable, tumor tissue. Clausen et al. (14) found ^{67}Ga localized primarily in the nuclear fraction of tumor tissue, while Anghileri (15) demonstrated ^{67}Ga binding to intracellular lipoproteins, nucleoproteins, phospholipids, and nucleic acids. The localization of ^{67}Ga has been likened to the localization of calcium and magnesium, with the speculation that ^{67}Ga displaces these ions from their intracellular divalent cation-binding sites (16,17). There is controversy over the relationship of ^{67}Ga accumulation, lesion growth rate, and metabolic activity. Some lesions clearly show a correlation between growth rate and ^{67}Ga uptake, whereas others do not (18–22). Considering the confusing array of observations, it is not surprising that few investigators agree on a single concept to explain the mechanism of ^{67}Ga localization.

LOCALIZATION IN NORMAL TISSUES

We have recently demonstrated that ^{67}Ga in human colostrum is bound primarily to lactoferrin (23). Lactoferrin is a protein with a molecular weight of approximately 80,000 and is somewhat similar in configuraation to transferrin. It binds both iron and gallium more avidly than transferrin and is therefore capable of attracting ^{67}Ga from transferrin. The migration of ^{67}Ga from transferrin to lactoferrin occurs most efficiently in an acid environment since ^{67}Ga binding to transferrin is inhibited below pH 7 while binding to lactoferrin is not inhibited above pH 3 to 4. Lactoferrin is present in high concentration in many of the normal tissues and secretions in which gallium localizes including lacrimal glands, tears, salivary glands, nasopharynx, spleen, bone marrow and gut. Lactoferrin is also a major protein constituent of neutrophilic leukocytes (24). Both lactoferrin and transferrin are metabolized in the liver. The combination of migration of ^{67}Ga from plasma proteins, principally transferrin, to tissue and secretory proteins such as lactoferrin as well as the normal metabolic accumulation and destruction of both transferrin and lactoferrin in the liver provides a convenient explanation of the normal pattern of ^{67}Ga localization.

LOCALIZATION IN INFLAMMATORY LESIONS

Gallium-67 localization in inflammatory disease is mediated in some way through the action of the neutrophilic leukocytes. [67]Ga uptake in abscesses is suppressed in severe leukopenia (25). It is unknown whether ^{67}Ga binds to leukocytes which subsequently migrate to the inflammatory lesion or the ^{67}Ga binds to leukocytes which have already localized in the lesion. Both mechanisms are possible. [67]Ga accumulation in such sites is enhanced by increased blood supply and the "leaky" capillary endothelium usually associated with both abscesses and tumors. Tsan and associates have shown that ^{67}Ga may also be taken up directly by many microorganisms. (26)

A number of possible explanations of the precise mechanism of ^{67}Ga localization exist. The ^{67}Ga-transferrin molecule may bind to the surface of both leukocytes and bacteria (transferrin is known to bind to cell surfaces) (27). Alternatively, ^{67}Ga either bound to transferrin or in the ionic state may pass into the cell and be protein-bound to intracellular proteins such as lactoferrin. Finally, ^{67}Ga may become incorporated into the leukocyte or bacteria as part of a metabolic enzyme system. The presence of lactoferrin in high concentration in neutrophilic leukocytes and the presence of this protein in abscess fluid suggests that it plays some role in the process.

LOCALIZATION IN TUMOR

Ito et al. (13) and Winchell and coworkers (28,29) postulate that ^{67}Ga is taken up in tumors as a result of binding to intracellur tumor proteins which compete successfully with transferrin for ^{67}Ga. Clausen and coworkers (14) showed that one-third of intracellular tumor ^{67}Ga is bound to ferritin. Ferritin is present in high concentration in certain malignancies such as Hodgkins disease as well as normal liver, spleen, gastrointestinal mucosa and bone marrow. Hayes and associates have found ^{67}Ga bound to 45,000 molecular weight glycoprotein in tumors (30).

Lactoferrin is also present in increased concentration in some tumors (32) although it has not been shown to bind ^{67}Ga within tumor. The exact mechanism by which ^{67}Ga enters the tumor cell to become associated with tumor proteins is unknown. It may diffuse in directly in ionic form, become attached to the cell surface in the form of ^{67}Ga-transferrin or ^{67}Ga-lactoferrin or be carried into the tumor region associated with inflammatory cellular elements.

GENERAL CONCLUSIONS

Most of the currently popular proposed mechanisms of ^{67}Ga localization assume that ^{67}Ga acts in part as an iron analog. It binds to iron binding proteins although it is incapable of becoming incorporated into the heme molecule, perhaps because of its inability to undergo reduction and subsequent reoxidation reactions within the body. Transferrin appears to act primarily as a carrier protein for ^{67}Ga, transporting it from the site of injection to the site of cellular localization. Greater knowledge about specific tissue proteins which are capable of ^{67}Ga binding may lead to improved radiopharmaceuticals for both tumor and abscess localization. Such proteins may be responsible for the localization of other cations as well.

REFERENCES

1. Hartman RE, Hayes RL: The binding of gallium by blood serum. *J Pharmacol Exp Ther* 168, 193, 1969.
2. Hartman RE, Hayes RL: Gallium binding by blood serum [Abstract]. *Fed Proc* **26**:780, 1967.
3. Gunasekera SW, King LJ, Lavender PJ: The behavior of tracer gallium-67 towards serum proteins. *Clin Chim Acta* **39**:401, 1972.

4. Oster ZH, Larson SM, Wagner HN Jr: Possible enhancement of ^{67}Ga-citrate imaging by iron dextran. *J Nucl Med* **17**:356, 1976.

5. Hayes RL, Edwards CL: The effect of stable scandium on red blood cells and on the retention and excretion of [67]gallium in humans [Abstract]. *South Med J* **66**:1339, 1973.

6. Hayes RL, Byrd BL, Carlton JE, et al: Effect of scandium on the distribution of ^{67}Ga in tumor-bearing animals [Abstract]. *J Nucl Med* **12**:437, 1971.

7. Edwards CL, Hayes RL: Tumor detection with 67-gallium citrate. Symposium 4, First World Federation of Biology and Nuclear Medicine, Tokyo, 1974.

8. Watson EE, Cloutier RJ, Gibbs WD: Whole-body retention of ^{67}Ga-citrate. *J Nucl Med* **14**:840, 1973.

9. Nelson B, Hayes RL, Edwards CL, et al: Distribution of gallium in human tissues after intravenous administration. *J Nucl Med* **13**:92, 1972.

10. Swartzendruber DC, Nelson B, Hayes RL: Gallium-67 localization in lysosomal-like granules of leukemic and nonleukemic murine tissues. *J Nat Cancer Inst* **46**:941, 1971.

11. Aulbert E, Gebhardt A, Schulz E, et al: Mechanism of ^{67}Ga accumulation in normal rat liver lysosomes. *Nucl-Med* **15**:185, 1976.

12. Brown DH, Byrd BL, Carlton JE, et al: A quantitative study of the subcellular localization of [67]Ga. *Cancer Res* **36**:956, 1976.

13. Ito Y, Okuyama S, Sato K, et al: [67]Ga tumor scanning and its mechanisms studied in rabbits. *Radiology* **100**:357, 1971.

14. Clausen J, Edeling C-J, Fogh J: [67]Ga binding to human serum proteins and tumor components. *Cancer Res* **34**:1931, 1974.

15. Anghileri LB: The mechanism of accumulation of radiogallium and radioanthanides in tumors. *J Nucl Biol Med* **17**:177, 1973.

16. Anghileri LB: On the similarity of alkaline earths metabolism and ^{67}Ga accumulation by liver as revealed by acute thioacetamide intoxication. *J Nucl Biol Med* **19**:145, 1975.

17. Anghileri LJ: Studies on the relationship between ^{67}Ga-citrate accumulation and calcium metabolism in tumor cells. *Nucl-Med* **12**:257, 1973.

18. Bichel P, Hansen HH: The incorporation of ^{67}Ga in normal and malignant cells and its dependence on growth rate. *Brit J Radiol* **45**:182, 1972.

19. Merz T, McKusick KA, Malmud LS, et al: Enhanced ^{67}Ga accumulation in lymphocytes stimulated by phytohemagglutinin [Abstract]. *J Nucl Med* **14**:428, 1973.

20. Otten JA, Tyndall RL, Estes PC, et al: Localization of gallium-67 during embryogenesis. *Proc Soc Exp Biol Med* **142**:92, 1973.

21. Orii H: Tumor scanning with gallium (^{67}Ga) and its mechanism studied in rats. *Strahlentherapie* **144**:192, 1972.

22. Hammersley PAG, Taylor DM: ^{67}Ga-citrate incorporation and DNA synthesis in tumors, in Radiopharmaceuticals, Subramanian G, Rhodes BA, Cooper JF, et al (eds), New York, Society of Nuclear Medicine, 1975, p. 447.

23. Hoffer PB, Huberty JP, Khayam-Bashi H: The association of ^{67}Ga and lactoferrin. *J Nucl Med,* **18**:713, 1977.

24. Masson PL, Heremans JF, Schonne E: Lactoferrin, an iron-binding protein ni [sic] neutrophilic leukocytes. *J Exp Med* **130**:643, 1969.

25. Gelrud LG, Arseneau JC, Milder MS, et al: The kinetics of [67]gallium incorporation into inflammatory lesions: experimental and clinical studies. *J Lab Clin Med* **83**:489, 1974.

26. Tsan MF, Chen WY, Scheffel U: Mechanism of gallium localization in inflammatory lesions. *J Nucl Med* **18**:619, 1977.

27. Stephton RG, Harris AW: Gallium-67 citrate uptake by cultured tumor cells, stimulated by serum transferrin. *J Nat Cancer Inst* **54**:1263, 1974.

28. Winchell HS: Mechanisms for localization of radiopharmaceuticals in neoplasms. *Sem Nucl Med* **6**:371, 1976.

29. Winchell HS, Sanchez PD, Watanabe CK, et al: Visualization of tumors in humans using ^{67}Ga-citrate and the Anger whole-body scanner, scintillation camera and tomographic scanner. *J Nucl Med* **11**:459, 1970.

30. Hayes RL, Carlton JE: A study of macromolecular binding of ^{67}Ga in normal and malignant animal tissue. *Cancer Res* **33**:3265, 1973.

31. Hayes RL: The tissue distribution of gallium radionuclides. *J Nucl Med* **18**:740, 1977.

32. Loisillier F, Got R, Burtin P, et al: Recherches sur la localisation tissulair et l'autoantigenicite de la lactotransferrine. *Protides Biol Fluids* **14**:133, 1966.

2
Imaging Technique

Paul B. Hoffer, M.D.

Professor of Diagnostic Radiology
Director, Section of Nuclear Medicine
Yale University School of Medicine
New Haven, Connecticut

Proper imaging of gallium-67 (^{67}Ga) is a technical challenge that has received inadequate attention. Because ^{67}Ga has a relatively short physical half-life and no particulate emissions, it can be administered in millicurie amounts. With most commonly used radionuclides, this advantage virtually assures that high-quality images will be obtained. However, ^{67}Ga emits a complex spectrum of γ rays that greatly complicate the task of imaging. The problem of obtaining good images is further complicated by localization of the radionuclide in the bowel. Indeed, the slow clinical acceptance of ^{67}Ga is probably due in large part to the poor quality of images obtained by use of some of the current techniques.

Gallium-67 is usually cyclotron produced by proton bombardment of an enriched zinc-68 ([68]Zn) target, resulting in a p, 2n reaction (1,2). It decays by electron capture and has a half-life of 78 hours. Its major photon emissions are summarized in Table 1 (3,4).

The goal in ^{67}Ga imaging is to achieve greatest photopeak sensitivity while minimizing acceptance of scattered radiation. An ideal ^{67}Ga imaging device should be capable of detecting the 93, 185, and 300 keV peaks of [67]Ga. Because most currently available instruments omit one or more of the ^{67}Ga peaks, each peak will be discussed separately.

The 93 keV photon emission of ^{67}Ga is the most abundant, and virtually 100% is absorbed in the thin, ½-in. sodium iodide (NaI) crystal of the Anger camera or the thicker 2-in. NaI crystal of the rectilinear scanner. Imaging with this photopeak does present problems. It is lowest man on the totem pole of energies. Therefore, a window set to include the 93 keV peak will also include considerable down-scatter from the higher-energy peaks. Scatter may arise from within the crystal or within the patient. In either case, it has a detrimental effect on the quality of the image produced with this energy window. The scatter problem is compounded by the fact that 93-keV photons, when undergoing scatter interactions, experience only minimal energy degradation. Therefore, the 93 keV photopeak must live not only in the shadow of scatter from higher-energy photopeaks but also in the shadow of its own scatter. The 93 keV photon also produces, within the crystal, the least light of any of the ^{67}Ga photopeaks. This causes poor energy resolution and compounds the problem of scatter rejection. When an Anger camera is used for imaging, the low light output from the crystal limits the spatial resolution at this energy. The problem of poor spatial resolution at low photon energies is especially troublesome with older Anger cameras.

TABLE 1   PHOTOPEAKS AND ABUNDANCE OF EMISSIONS OF
            [67]Ga*

Energy (keV)	Abundance per 100 Disintegrations
93[†]	41
185	23
300	18
394	4

*After data of Dillman and Van der Lage (3) and of Martin (4).
[†]Includes 91 keV peak with three photons per 100 disintegrations.

Despite all of the deficiencies of the 93 keV peak, it is still the most important γ emission for ^{67}Ga imaging. Although the energy of the 93-keV photon is below the optimal imaging range, it is still acceptable. Furthermore, recent improvements in intrinsic resolution of the Anger camera have most dramatically affected imaging with photons in the 100 keV range.

The 185 keV photopeak is present in intermediate abundance. Although it too is contaminated by down-scatter from higher-energy photons, the problem of down-scatter is less severe than with the 93 keV peak. Spatial resolution for the 185 keV photon is excellent when the Anger camera is used. When triple windowing is employed, this photon contributes about 25% of the photopeak events.

The 300 keV photopeak is relatively free from the effect of down-scatter. Its high energy does, however, diminish relative detection efficiency when thin crystals are used. If triple windowing is employed, the 300 keV peak contributes about 25% of detected photopeak events with a 2-in. thick crystal (as in the dual probe scanner) but only about 10% of photopeak events with a ½-in. crystal (Anger camera).

The 394 keV photopeak is so high in energy and low in abundance that major efforts to employ it for imaging are not worthwhile. Even if detection of this photon were attempted, the photon would only contribute 2% of total detected counts with a ½-in. thick crystal and 3% of detected counts with a 2-in. thick crystal. Nevertheless, the 394 keV photopeak must not be totally disregarded, because it plays a major role in collimator selection.

SINGLE-PEAK VERSUS MULTIPLE-PEAK IMAGING

Gallium-67 images are almost always severely limited by the number of detected events used to construct the image. Therefore, every attempt must be made to improve the statistical content of the image. No single peak contributes more than 50–60% of the total potential data obtainable when all photopeak events from the 93, 185, and 300 keV peaks are collected. Therefore, the advantage of detecting multiple peaks is obvious. However, single-window detectors, that is, devices with only one pulse-height analyzer, do not usually allow detection of more than one photopeak. Furthermore, inclusion of more than one photopeak in a broad single window may create as many problems as it solves.

When only a single photopeak can be imaged, it is preferable to use the 93 keV peak, because it contains about as many photons as the 185 keV peak and the 300 keV peak combined. However, there are special circumstances (e.g., when an extremely obese patient is being evaluated or an older model Anger camera is used) in which a higher-energy photon is preferable for imaging. It must be emphasized that selection of the 93 keV photon for imaging does *not* imply use of a low-energy collimator.

SINGLE WIDE WINDOW VERSUS MULTIPLE WINDOWS

Most rectilinear scanners can be converted to accept two, three, or even four of the ^{67}Ga photon energies in a single pulse-height analyszer window (5,6). The advantage of such a wide window is that it achieves maximum counting efficiency. The disadvantage is that a large amount of scattered radiation is detected. A wide window detects not only the multiple photopeaks but also the broad valleys between the peaks. These valleys are inhabited almost exclusively by scattered radiation. Scatter degrades the quality of the image. If the statistical quality of the image is very poor, acceptance of some scattered radiation is the price paid for improvement in count density. However, as count density increases, acceptance of scattered radiation becomes less desirable.

A good rule of thumb (and it is only that) is to attempt to maintain a count density of at least 200 counts per square centimeter over the liver. If this density requires a broad window, it should be used. As a count density of 200 counts per square centimeter is achieved, the width of the window should be decreased to include fewer peaks and less scatter. Since the 93 keV peak is the most abundant, it acts as an anchor on a sliding peak scale. The window should be narrowed by eliminating the 394, the 300, and the 185 keV peaks in that order.*

A preferred approach is to modify the scanning unit with two additional pulse-height analyzers for each detector. The 93, 185, and 300 keV peaks can then be windowed separately. Although each such window includes some scattered radiation from higher peaks, the scatter valleys are eliminated. With use of such a modified scanner and a 3–5 mCi dose of ^{67}Ga citrate, count densities of 250 counts per square centimeter or higher can be achieved in total-body scan times of 1 hour or less (Figure 1) (8).

A comprehensive evaluation of photopeak selection for ^{67}Ga imaging with the

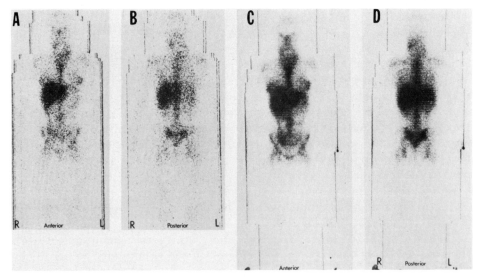

Figure 1.   Gallium-67 images obtained 72 hours after injection on the same patient with single, 185 keV peak window (A and B) and three separate windows bracketing the 93, 185, and 300 keV peaks (C and D). The marked improvement in image quality obtained with the triple window is due primarily to the fourfold increase in count density. This patient had cervical and iliac node involvement by lymphoma, in addition to slight breast uptake of [67]Ga.

*Harris (7) believes that the scatter region between the 93 and 185 keV peaks is so detrimental to image quality that all multipeak single windows should not include this range. It is difficult to get any consensus on an ideal single window.

dual 5-in. scanner was made by Ross and associates in 1971 (9). Their investigation evidently served as the basis for pulse-height analyzer window selection in the Oak Ridge "Cooperative Group" clinical study of gallium imaging. A single window that included the 185 and 300 keV gallium peaks was used in that study, and some investigators have inferred that it is the optimal window for ^{67}Ga imaging. But, in fact, the Oak Ridge study found the optimal method of ^{67}Ga imaging to be the use of four separate pulse-height analyzers, one for each major gallium peak. The 185–300 keV single window produced only marginally better images than did a single 93–185 keV window, and then only if the worst condition of maximum scatter was assumed. A novel finding was that by using only two pulse-height analyzers, one for the 93 keV peak and one for the 185, 300, and 394 keV peaks combined, good results could be achieved.

With the conventional Anger camera, window flexibility is considerably reduced. Few of the Anger cameras in current use have more than one pulse-height analyzer. Older versions of the camera that are equipped with two pulse-height analyzers show considerable degradation in resolution when the two windows are used simultaneously. This problem has been corrected in most multiple-window cameras manufactured since 1975.

It is not possible, with even the widest single window, to include more than one peak within the window of an Anger camera equipped with a single pulse-height analyzer. This is just as well, since a broader window that includes multiple peaks of widely differing energies would produce significant field nonuniformity. As previously noted, the 93 keV peak is usually the optimum choice when the Anger camera is used for imaging ^{67}Ga because of its greater detection efficiency. A symmetric 20 or 25% window should be used to bracket the peak.

Twenty percent windows about the photopeak are usually suitable when a separate pulse-height analyzer is used for each peak in combination with either a rectilinear scanner or a newer type of multiwindow camera. Some investigators advocate slightly wider windows, but the differences are marginal. If more than one photopeak is included in the window, a much wider and asymmetric window is, of course, required.

CHOICE OF COLLIMATOR

The most significant common technical error in performing ^{67}Ga scans is the use of an inappropriate collimator. The correct collimator is determined not by the energy of the γ ray to be imaged but by the highest-energy photon emitted by the radionuclide *within the patient.*

When a thin-septa (low energy) collimator is used in association with a gamma emitter that has both high- and low-energy emissions, the collimator is a more efficient attenuator for the low-energy photons than for the high-energy photons. This is largely because of the greater septal penetration that occurs in thin-septa collimators with high-energy photons. On the crystal side of the collimator, the effect of this septal penetration is a high ratio of uncollimated high-energy photons to collimated low-energy photons. This, in itself, is not detrimental, because when the lower-energy photons are windowed, the higher-energy photon-crystal interactions should be rejected. However, the crystal is an imperfect absorber of high-energy photons. Many of the high-energy photons deposit only part of their energy in the crystal in the process of being scattered. Therefore, even a narrow low-energy window will be heavily contaminated by an abundance of low-energy pulses resulting from scattering and partial energy absorption of essentially uncollimated high-energy photons by the crystal. The net effect is marked degradation of image quality. A collimator with thicker septa, designed to have minimal septal penetration for the 394 keV photons, will have the same ratio of high- to low-energy photons on the crystal side of the collimator as on the patient side. Although crystal scatter can also occur in this situation, there are proportionally fewer high-energy photons to scatter, and even these events are appropriately collimated. These points are illustrated in Figure 2.

CHOICE OF INSTRUMENT

Often the choice of instruments to perform a specific imaging task, such as a ^{67}Ga citrate scan, is dictated by availability rather than by suitability. Almost any dual 5-in. scanner or Anger camera can be used to produce reasonable ^{67}Ga images, provided that both proper technique and an appropriate radionuclide dose and collimator are used. Instrument selection should be determined to a large extent on the basis of efficiency. The most efficient system, a large-field (15 in. diameter) Anger camera with triple-window capability, is about eight times more efficient than the least efficient system, a dual 5-in. scanner with a single 93 keV peak window.

If an inherently low-efficiency system must be used, special effort should be made to improve the statistical quality of the image. The maximum permissible radionuclide dose should be used; the imaging should be restricted to the region of specific interest, if there is one; and the imaging time should be as long as possible, that is, consistent with patient comfort. Few patients can tolerate scan times beyond 1 hour.

Background subtraction or contrast enhancement may be useful in interpreting rectilinear scans with moderate count densities. Such techniques, however, do not improve the statistical quality of a low count image and are often unnecessary on higher count images.

If total-body imaging is desired, for example, in staging of Hodgkin's disease, a reasonably high-efficiency system must be employed to achieve optimum diagnostic results. In some situations, slight sacrifice in efficiency may be indicated if some other benefit is to be achieved. For example, although the Anger tomoscanner is not as efficient as the Anger large-field camera, the advantage of having a tomographic readout may outweigh a slight sacrifice in sensitivity. Examples of images from both a large-field camera and a tomoscanner are shown in Figures 3 and 4.

Experienced clinicians make more accurate diagnoses from images obtained with a large-field (15 in. diameter) Anger camera equipped with three pulse-height analyzers than from those obtained with a lower-efficiency single pulse-height analyzer, dual 5-in. rectilinear scanner (10) (Figure 5).

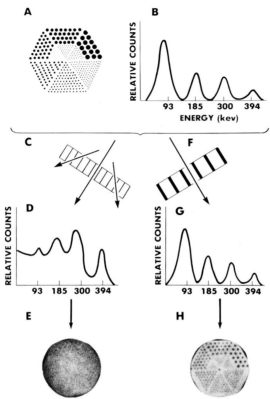

Figure 2.   The effect of a thin, as compared with a thick, septa collimator on ^{67}Ga images obtained
with an Anger camera and 20% window peaked at 93 keV and with an Anger cold-spot phantom.
The phantom (A) consists of Lucite cylinders (seen on end) of various diameters surrounded by a
solution of ^{67}Ga. The relative intensity of the four major photon peaks being emitted from the
phantom is also illustrated (B). A thin-septa low-energy collimator (C) lets many of the higher-energy
photons pass into the detector inadequately collimated and relatively less attenuated than the lower-
energy photons. The resultant spectrum from the detector (D) shows an increase in abundance of
higher-energy photons relative to low-energy photons. The lower-energy peaks are not only relatively diminished but also ride on a high background of down-scatter that results from incomplete
absorption of high-energy photons by the detector. Therefore, even when the 93 keV peak is used
for imaging, a poor-quality image is obtained (E). However, when a thicker-septa middle- or high-
energy collimator (F) is used, all photons are collimated and attenuated equally. Less down-scatter
occurs, and the spectral distribution of photons seen by the detector (G) as a result of collimation is
virtually unchanged. The diminution of crystal scatter events compared to 93 keV photopeak events
results in a good-quality image (H). Remember, the energy spectrum of the activity within the patient
dictates collimator selection, *not* the photopeak or window selected for imaging.

PATIENT PREPARATION

Colonic activity can cause confusion in detection of intra-abdominal lesions on
gallium scans. For unknown reasons, the amount of bowel activity is highly
variable. Most colonic activity is within the bowel lumen; therefore, bowel preparation by use of an evacuant or enema or both has been advocated. While there

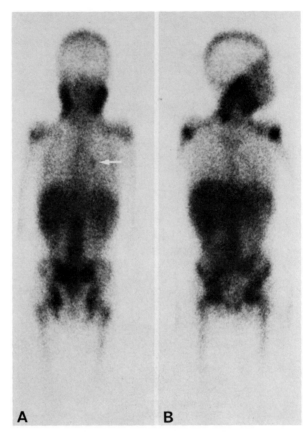

Figure 3.   Gallium-67 citrate scan obtained with a large-field camera with triple window and moving table; anterior (A) and posterior (B) views. The patient was a child with Hodgkin's disease who had bronchial obstruction due to a mediastinal mass. Two thousand rads were delivered to a thoracic midline port to relieve obstruction while the exact extent of the disease was being determined. The scan reveals bilateral cervical node involvement and also diminished activity in the mediastinal component of the tumor and in the portion of the thoracic spine included in the radiation port. A small pericardial lesion (arrow) was also detected beyond the margin of the radiation port and might otherwise have escaped treatment if a less sensitive or lower-resolution imaging system had been used.

is evidence that bowel preparation is ineffective in eliminating the colonic activity (11), most clinicians still use it because they believe that it does decrease the amount of bowel activity seen on scan.

A commonly used method of bowel preparation is the administration of laxatives, such as 15 mg of bisacodyl (Dulcolax), orally each day, starting on the day of injection of the radionuclide and continuing until imaging is completed. For postoperative scans, 12 oz (360 ml) of citrate of magnesia is administered on the evening prior to the initial scan. If significant bowel activity is observed on the 48- or 72-hour postinjection images, an enema is given and the scan is repeated on the next day.

Patients should not be denied a gallium scan because their clinical condition

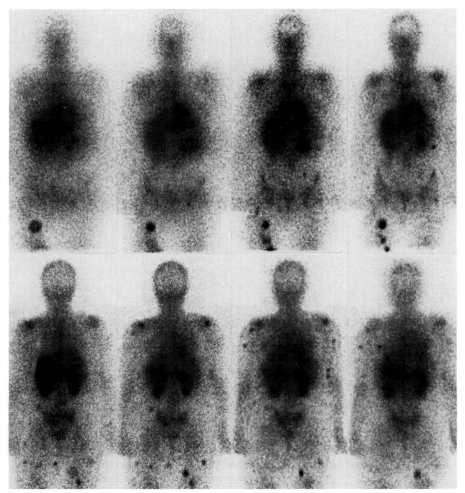

Figure 4.   Gallium-67 scan obtained with the Anger tomoscanning device. The patient was a 44-year-old woman who had had a melanoma resected, then returned for evaluation of a small subcutaneous nodule in the left arm above the elbow. The tomoscan demonstrates multiple areas of involvement, including the heart. The multiple focal plane images allow determination of the exact location of each lesion. (Courtesy of Dr. Ernest Fordham, Department of Nuclear Medicine, Presbyterian-St. Luke's Health Center, Chicago, Illinois.)

precludes vigorous bowel preparation. In such patients, the usual preparation should be withheld, but the imaging should be performed anyway. In some of these patients, no bowel activity will be seen; in others, bowel activity will not seriously interfere with interpretation of the scan. In situations in which bowel activity does interfere with interpretation and the use of enemas or evacuants is contraindicated, a scan performed 1 or 2 days after the first scan will often show clearing of the activity from the bowel or some movement of the activity along the path of the colon. Focal areas of activity in the region of the colon that do not move or decrease in intensity within a few days are probably not within the bowel lumen.

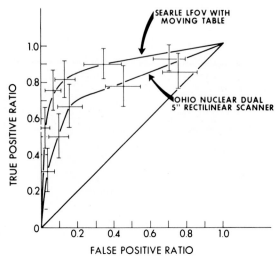

Figure 5.   Receiver operating characteristic curves comparing mean performance among four experienced observers reading scans obtained with a single window (93 and 185 keV peaks), dual, 5-in. rectilinear scanner and a large field of view (LFOV) camera with triple window and moving table. The better performance of all four observers using the large field camera was due to the higher sensitivity of the camera and to improved scatter rejection by means of multiple, separate windows. The differences in performance were statistically significant, as determined by a paired-sample comparison.

IMAGING TIMES

Most gallium scans for evaluation and staging of malignancy should be performed approximately 72 hours after injection of the radionuclide. At 72 hours, the rapid phase of blood pool clearance of gallium has been completed, and the gallium in the colon has had an opportunity to be evacuated. The period between injection and imaging can be shortened to 48 hours or extended to 96 or 120 hours without serious compromise of lesion detectability. Usually a single set of images is adequate. However, if bowel activity persists, scanning can be repeated the next day, after additional bowel preparation. On rare occasions, a second, 24-hour delayed scan must be obtained.

Recommendations for imaging inflammatory lesions are presented in chapter 6. In general, an initial scan is obtained within the first 24 hours after injection of the radionuclide. If a lesion cannot be definitely identified, a repeat scan is obtained at either 48 or 72 hours.

VIEWS

The choice of regions imaged and views obtained depends on the indications for performing the procedure. At least one set of whole-body scans is helpful, but it should not be obtained when the region of the suspected disease is known and the instrument available for imaging cannot produce a high count-density total-body image in a short time. Lateral and oblique views of suspicious-looking regions are also sometimes helpful.

DECAY SCHEMES AND DOSIMETRY DATA

The exact decay scheme and radiation input and output data for ^{67}Ga are included in Figure 6. These data, from MIRD pamphlet 10 (3), have since been modified by more recent information about the abundance of the major imaging

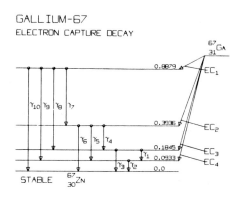

```
         ..INPUT DATA..

   31 GALLIUM 67        HALF LIFE = 78.1 HOURS

   DECAY MODE- ELECTRON CAPTURE
   ------------------------------------------
                   MEAN      TRAN-
                   NUMBER/   SITION    OTHER
                   DISINTE-  ENERGY    NUCLEAR
   TRANSITION      GRATION   (MEV)     DATA
   ------------------------------------------
   ELECT CAPT  1   0.0033    0.1170    ALLOWED
   ELECT CAPT  2   0.2290    0.6110    ALLOWED
   ELECT CAPT  3   0.2520    0.8200    ALLOWED
   ELECT CAPT  4   0.5157    0.9120    ALLOWED
      GAMMA    1   0.0351    0.0913    M1, AK= 0.0660
                                       AL= 0.00760
      GAMMA    2   0.7135    0.0933    E2, AK= 0.770
                                       K/M=58.0
                                       AL= 0.100
      GAMMA    3   0.2420    0.1846    M1, AK= 0.0156
                                       K/M=65.0
                                       AL= 0.00170
      GAMMA    4   0.0250    0.2090    M1, AK= 0.00750
                                       K/L=10.6
                                       K/M=61.0
      GAMMA    5   0.1620    0.3002    M1, AK= 0.00337
                                       K/L= 9.50
                                       K/M=75.0
      GAMMA    6   0.0430    0.3936    M1, AK= 0.00192
                                       AL(T) =
                                       0.000144
      GAMMA    7   0.0010    0.4943    M1, AK= 0.00119
                                       AL(T) =
                                       0.000085
      GAMMA    8   0.0001    0.7036    M1,  AK(T) =
                                       0.000461
                                       AL(T) =
                                       0.000039
      GAMMA    9   0.0006    0.7947    M1,  AK(T) =
                                       0.000354
                                       AL(T) =
                                       0.000030
      GAMMA   10   0.0015    0.8880    M1, AK=0.000337
                                       AL(T) =
                                       0.000024

   ------------
   REF.- LI-SCHOLZ, A. AND BAKHRU, H., PHYS. REV.
       1778 1629 (1969).
       FREEDMAN, M.S. ET AL, PHYS. REV. 151, 886
       (1966).
```

```
         ..OUTPUT DATA..

   31 GALLIUM 67        HALF LIFE = 78.1 HOURS

   DECAY MODE- ELECTRON CAPTURE
   ------------------------------------------
                       MEAN      MEAN     EQUI-
                       NUMBER/   ENERGY/  LIBRIUM
                       DISINTE-  PAR-     DOSE
   RADIATION           GRATION   TICLE    CONSTANT

                         n_i       Ē_i      Δ_i
                                  (MEV)    (g-rad/
                                           μCi-h)
   ------------------------------------------
        GAMMA     1     0.0326    0.0913    0.0063
   K INT CON ELECT     0.0021    0.0816    0.0003
        GAMMA     2     0.3797    0.0933    0.0754
   K INT CON ELECT     0.2830    0.0836    0.0504
   L INT CON ELECT     0.0379    0.0922    0.0074
   M INT CON ELECT     0.0126    0.0932    0.0025
        GAMMA     3     0.2388    0.1846    0.0939
   K INT CON ELECT     0.0026    0.1749    0.0009
   L INT CON ELECT     0.0004    0.1835    0.0001
        GAMMA     4     0.0247    0.2090    0.0110
        GAMMA     5     0.1613    0.3002    0.1031
   K INT CON ELECT     0.0005    0.2905    0.0003
        GAMMA     6     0.0429    0.3936    0.0359
        GAMMA     7     0.0009    0.4943    0.0010
        GAMMA     8     0.0001    0.7036    0.0002
        GAMMA     9     0.0006    0.7947    0.0010
        GAMMA    10     0.0015    0.8880    0.0029
   K ALPHA-1 X-RAY     0.3075    0.0086    0.0056
   K ALPHA-2 X-RAY     0.1534    0.0086    0.0028
   K BETA-1 X-RAY      0.0553    0.0095    0.0011
   KLL AUGER ELECT     0.5185    0.0075    0.0083
   KLX AUGER ELECT     0.1410    0.0085    0.0025
   KXY AUGER ELECT     0.0067    0.0094    0.0001
   LMM AUGER ELECT     1.7722    0.0008    0.0033
   MXY AUGER ELECT     3.7779    0.0000    0.0006
```

*From MIRD Pamphlet 10 (3).

Figure 6. Decay scheme and radiation input and radiation output data for ^{67}Ga. [From Dillman and Van der Lage (3).]

TABLE 2   ESTIMATED ABSORBED DOSE
FROM A SINGLE INTRAVENOUS
INJECTION OF RADIOGALLIUM CITRATE (^{67}Ga)*

Tissue	Rads per Millicurie Injected
Stomach	0.22
Small intestine	0.36
Upper large intestine	0.56
Lower large intestine	0.90
Gonads	
Ovaries	0.28
Testes	0.24
Kidneys	0.41
Liver	0.46
Marrow	0.58
Skeleton	0.44
Spleen	0.53
Total body	0.26

*Based on MIRD dose estimate report 2 (12).

photon emissions (4). They are included for convenience in calculating radiation doses from ^{67}Ga. Radiation dose estimates are presented in Table 2 and are based on MIRD dose estimate report 2 (12). The calculations of radiation dose to the gut were probably overestimated in that report, because the biologic data were obtained from subjects who did not undergo bowel cleansing procedures.

SUMMARY OF TECHNICAL CONSIDERATIONS IN ^{67}Ga IMAGING

Information density is critical and should be greater than 200 counts per square centimeter over the liver. If an image with this information density cannot be achieved in a reasonable scanning time, consider the following modifications: restricting the field to be imaged and using the imaging time to detect more counts from this smaller region, or widening the window to include more peaks, or both.

A middle- or high-energy collimator *must* be used for ^{67}Ga imaging, regardless of the type of imaging instrument or energy window selected for imaging. A collimator suitable for imaging iodine-131 (364 keV) is suitable for ^{67}Ga imaging. Most "middle-energy" collimators are adequate.

Technically optimal ^{67}Ga images require count densities in the range of 1000 counts per square centimeter over the liver and restriction of the scatter fraction component by means of separate windowing of the 93, 185, and 300 keV peaks, using 20% symmetric windows. The two instruments best suited for ^{67}Ga imaging are the large-field (15 in. diameter) Anger camera with multiple window selection and the Anger tomoscanner.

REFERENCES

1. Silvester DJ, Thakur, ML: Cyclotron production of carrier-free gallium-67,[Letter to the editor]. *Int J Appl Radiation Isotopes* **21**:630, 1970.

2. Porter J. Kawana M, Krizek H, et al: [67]Ga production with a compact cyclotron. *J Nucl Med* **11**:352, 1970.

3. Dillman LT, Van der Lage FC: Radionuclide decay schemes and nuclear parameters for use in radiation-dose estimation. MIRD pamphlet 10, New York, Society of Nuclear Medicine, 1975, p. 39.

4. Martin M: Nuclear decay data for selected nuclides. Oak Ridge National Laboratory Report 5114, 1976.

5. Yeh E-L: Simple way to widen the spectrometer window in the Ohio-nuclear scanner for ^{67}Ga scanning [Letter to the editor]. *J Nucl Med* **14**:361, 1973.

6. Cox RS, Turner DA, Fordham EW: Modification of a rectilinear scanner to improve ^{67}Ga scans. *J Nucl Med* **16**:1192, 1975.

7. Harris C: Personal communication, 1976.

8. Hoffer PB, Turner D, Gottschalk A, et al: Whole-body radiogallium scanning for staging of Hodgkin's disease and other lymphomas. *Nat Cancer Inst Monogr* **36**:277, 1973.

9. Ross DA, McClain WJ, East JK, et al: Multiple-window spectrometry for gallium-67. Oak Ridge National Laboratory Report, ORNL-TM-3260, 1971.

10. Hoffer PB, Schor RA, Ashby DA, et al: A comparison of ^{67}Ga-citrate images obtained with rectilinear scanner and large field Anger camera. *J Nucl Med.* in press.

11. Zeman R, Ryerson T: The value of bowel preparation in gallium-67 citrate scanning [Abstract] *J Nucl Med* **17**:559, 1976.

12. MIRD Dose Estimate Report 2, Summary of current radiation dose estimates to humans from [66]Ga-, [67]Ga-, [68]Ga-, and [72]Ga-citrate. *J Nucl Med* **14**:755, 1973.

3

Normal Patterns of Localization

Steven M. Larson, M.D.

Assistant Chief of Nuclear Medicine Section
Veterans Administration Hospital

Associate Professor of Medicine,
Laboratory Medicine, and Radiology
University of Washington
Seattle, Washington

Paul B. Hoffer, M.D.

Professor of Diagnostic Radiology
Director, Section of Nuclear Medicine
Yale University School of Medicine
New Haven, Connecticut

When carrier-free gallium-67 (^{67}Ga) citrate is injected intravenously, the majority of the radiopharmaceutical is quickly bound to plasma proteins, particularly transferrin (1). During the first 24 hours after intravenous administration, the kidney excretes about 10–25% of the administered dose. During this interval, the kidney and bladder may contain the highest concentration of radionuclide. After 24 hours, the fecal route of excretion predominates. About one third of the isotope is excreted over the first week, and the remaining two thirds are retained within the body tissues for prolonged periods (2). In autopsy studies, Nelson and associates (3) observed the following distribution of injected isotope within the body: liver, 2.8%/kg;* spleen, 4.1%/kg; kidney, 2.7%/kg; skeleton, including marrow, 2.5%/kg; and other soft tissues, less than 0.5%/kg. Other organs with a relatively high concentration of ^{67}Ga included the adrenals, bowel, and lungs. This distribution is somewhat different from that observed in clinical images, because it is based on data from terminally ill patients, obtained at a broad range of intervals after injection, and not all of the radionuclide was carrier free.

NORMAL ^{67}Ga IMAGE

The normal whole-body ^{67}Ga photoscan 72 hours after ^{67}Ga citrate intravenous injection is shown in Figure 1. There is prominent uptake in the liver and skeleton. Uptake in the colon, due to excretion of gallium into the gut, is also often seen at 72 hours. Activity in the kidneys, which may be observed at 24 hours, is no longer detectable. Prominent uptake is normally present in the nasal mucosa (best seen on the anterior projection) and in the region of the occiput (best noted on the posterior projection). The lacrimal glands concentrate ^{67}Ga and may be strikingly prominent on the anterior projection (4) (Figure 2). Uptake in the salivary glands is sometimes observed. In the thorax, ^{67}Ga is normally distributed within the rib cage, spine, and scapulae. Concentration of ^{67}Ga in the sternum may be prominent. At times, this uptake may be so active as to mimic tumor in the mediastinum. The triangular shape of the manubrium with the apex pointed downward is of some benefit in aiding one to differentiate the sternum from enlarged hilar or peritracheal lymph nodes.

Within the abdomen, in addition to the liver and spleen, uptake of gallium in the bowel, particularly the ascending and transverse colon, is frequently seen. This activity may persist despite repeated attempts at cleansing enemas. In the extremities, the concentration of ^{67}Ga is normally greatest in the epiphyseal regions of the long bones and is prominent in the shoulders, elbows, and knees.

The distribution of ^{67}Ga seen on the scan image depends to some extent on the interval between injection of the radionuclide and imaging. Gallium is cleared relatively slowly from the blood, so that by 24 hours, as much as 20% of the injected dose is still within the blood pool. This blood pool retention is reflected in the prominence of soft tissue activity on 6- and 24-hour scans. During the initial 24 hours, there is also rapid renal excretion, resulting in increased renal activity. In scans performed after 24 hours following injection,

* All values are percentage of injected dose per kilogram.

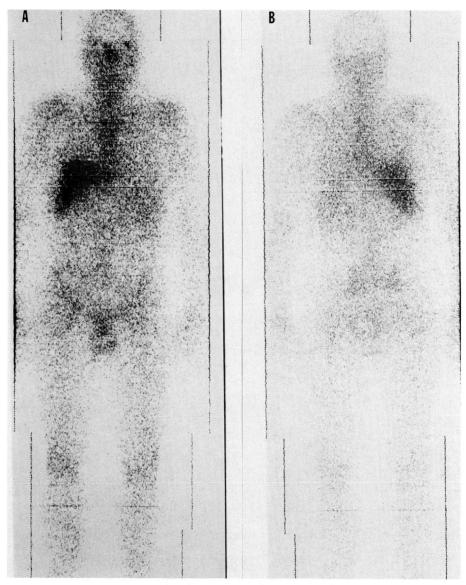

Figure 1.   Anterior (A) and posterior (B) rectilinear scan images obtained 72 hours after intraven-ous injection of ^{67}Ga citrate. Activity is most prominent in the liver and, to a lesser extent, in the bone and bone marrow. Lacrimal, nasopharyngeal, genital, and faint splenic activity are also seen, as is diffuse soft-tissue background activity. The relative distribution of activity in these normal sites of localization may vary considerably.

renal activity is rarely detectable, and the soft tissue uptake is less prominent. Figure 3 shows a normal image at 24 hours, with some renal uptake and consid-erable radioactivity accumulating in the bladder. By 48 and 72 hours, the dis-tribution of gallium within the body is very near an equilibrium state.

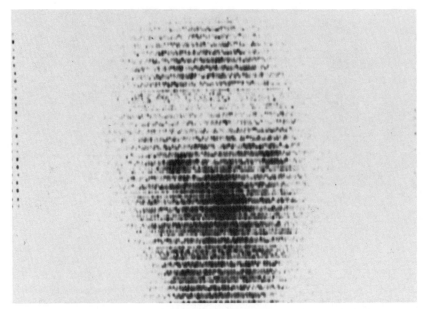

Figure 2.   Prominent activity in the lacrimal glands is seen on this anterior view of the head. Lacrimal activity was originally thought to be due to ^{67}Ga binding to transferrin, which is present in tears (4). It is likely that ^{67}Ga is also bound to lactoferrin, a somewhat similar protein, which is present in tears and has higher affinity for ^{67}Ga than does transferrin.

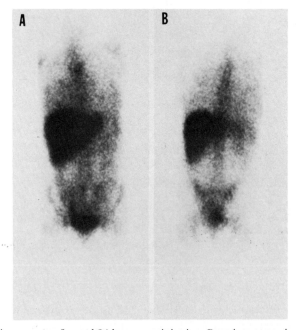

Figure 3.   Gallium scan performed 24 hours postinjection. Prominent anterior pelvic activity (A) is seen in the bladder and is frequently observed on scans performed within 24 hours of injection. The left kidney is also faintly seen on the posterior view (B). Moderate activity may also occasionally be seen diffusely throughout the lungs and abdomen on these early images, making it difficult to diagnose a diffuse pneumonia or peritonitis.

NORMAL VARIANTS

Bowel Uptake

The uptake of ^{67}Ga in the bowel may be very prominent, as is shown in Figure 4. This extent of uptake obscures the entire abdominal area and makes the interpretation of the gallium scan in the region of the abdomen virtually impossi-

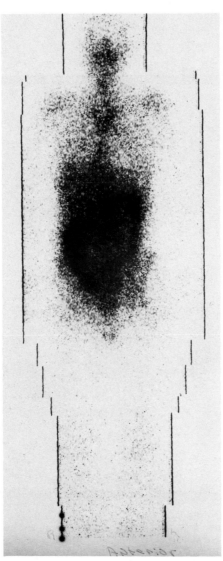

Figure 4.   Prominent bowel activity on anterior view obtained 72 hours after intravenous injection of ^{67}Ga citrate. The extent of bowel activity varies considerably. Most bowel activity is present within the colonic lumen and can be removed by adequate bowel preparation prior to scan. Some activity may, however, be localized in the colonic mucosa and will not clear completely, even after vigorous bowel preparation. In some patients, it may be difficult to distinguish normal bowel activity from the diffuse bowel localization of ^{67}Ga described in pseudomembranous colitis (11).

ble. More commonly, lesser degrees of colonic uptake are seen; often, only a portion of the bowel is visualized.

Occasionally, it is desirable to administer a nonabsorbable radionuclide, such as ^{99m}Tc-sulfur colloid, orally to identify the bowel and determine if activity seen on the gallium scan is intra- or extraluminal. Figure 5 shows scans of a 77-year-old woman with abdominal pain, in whom a prominent area of uptake is noted in the region of the left upper quadrant. Oral technetium sulfur colloid clearly outlines the stomach lumen. The gallium uptake is in close proximity to the stomach but not within its lumen. The patient proved to have a lymphoma infiltrating the gastric mucosa.

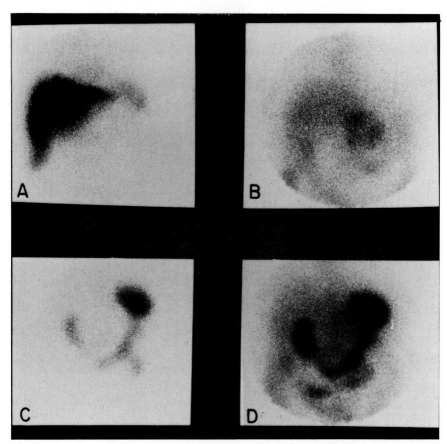

Figure 5.   Use of oral ^{99m}Tc-sulfur colloid in conjuction with a ^{67}Ga citrate scan to distinguish intraluminal from extraluminal ^{67}Ga activity. The anterior view of a prior liver scan (A) is normal in appearance in this 77-year-old patient with abdominal pain. The anterior view on the ^{67}Ga scan (B) demonstrates nonhepatic activity in the region of the stomach. Oral ^{99m}Tc-sulfur colloid was then administered, and the patient was reimaged in the same position (C), but with the 140 keV window for ^{99m}Tc (and a *middle*-energy collimator!). The stomach and proximal jejunum are clearly imaged. Superimposition of the ^{67}Ga and ^{99m}Tc-sulfur colloid images (D) reveals ^{67}Ga activity in a lesion medial to the stomach that proved at operation to be a lymphomatous mass infiltrating into the stomach wall.

Breast Uptake

Prominent uptake may occur in the breast, particularly when the breasts are under the physiologic stimulus of the menarche, cyclic estrogenic or progestational agents, or pregnancy (5). Figure 6 is a photoscan of a woman with

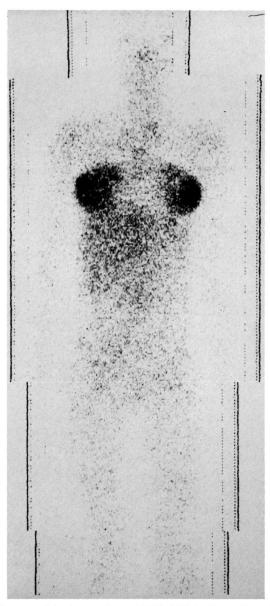

Figure 6.   Bilateral breast activity in a patient with Hodgkin's disease 3 weeks after birth of her infant. Gallium-67 concentrates in colostrum principally in association with lactoferrin. This iron-binding protein constitutes about 15% of the total protein in human milk and has the capacity to remove ^{67}Ga from transferrin due to its greater binding affinity. Though this patient was not lactating, her breasts did contain colostrum.

Hodgkin's disease who was scanned 3 weeks after the birth of her infant. The patient was not nursing, but she was able to manually express a small amount of milk from both breasts. The ^{67}Ga concentration was measured at 90 and 120 hours after injection and found to be 70 nCi per milliliter. Thus, ^{67}Ga in appreciable amounts was being excreted in milk.

Although ^{67}Ga uptake has been associated with both benign and malignant breast lesions, it also occurs in nonlactating women with no breast abnormalities, as seen in Figure 7. Therefore, faint ^{67}Ga localization in breast tissue should be considered a normal variant.

Hepatic Uptake

Liver uptake may vary on early views obtained within the first 24 hours postinjection but becomes progressively more prominent in most normal individuals on the 48- and 72-hour images. Faint or absent liver uptake often results from competing uptake by tumor or inflammation. Liver uptake may, however, be depressed by certain specific noninflammatory and nonmalignant processes. If

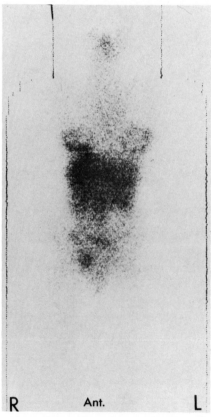

R   Ant.   L

Figure 7.   Faint asymmetric ^{67}Ga localization in the breasts of a nonlactating patient with Hodgkin's disease. The patient did have involvement of mesenteric and right inguinal lymph nodes, which also concentrated ^{67}Ga.

chemotherapeutic agents, such as vincristine, are administered within 24 hours of the injection of ^{67}Ga citrate, liver uptake is depressed. High levels of circulating iron will produce saturation of serum transferrin and also depress ^{67}Ga uptake in the liver. Hepatic failure will produce a similar pattern (Figure 8). When hepatic uptake is depressed by any of these factors, renal uptake will usually occur; the kidneys will remain prominent on images obtained at 72 hours or later.

A normal appearing distribution of ^{67}Ga in the liver does not exclude a hepatic lesion. Gallium is taken up by the normal liver with an avidity about equal to that of most pathologic lesions. When hepatic pathology is suspected, a ^{99m}Tc-sulfur colloid scan of the liver should be obtained. A lesion that is present on the ^{99m}Tc-sulfur colloid liver scan, that is, a region of decreased activity, and that "disappears" on the ^{67}Ga scan should be considered a gallium-positive lesion. The necessity for the colloid scan in properly interpreting ^{67}Ga uptake in the liver is demonstrated in Figure 9.

Salivary Gland Uptake

Prominent salivary gland uptake frequently occurs after irradiation of the neck (6) (Figure 10). This uptake is apparently due to radiation sialadenitis and must

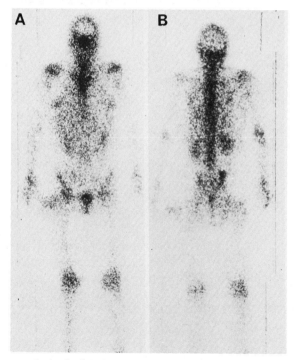

Figure 8.   Gallium uptake in the liver is markedly diminished (A), and renal activity (B) is prominent. This pattern can be seen in hepatic failure, diseases associated with elevated serum iron levels, and if gallium is injected within 24 hours of administration of certain chemotherapeutic agents, such as vincristine. In this case, the absence of hepatic uptake of gallium was due to acute hepatic failure. The ^{99m}Tc-sulfur colloid scan revealed virtually no colloid uptake in the liver (C).

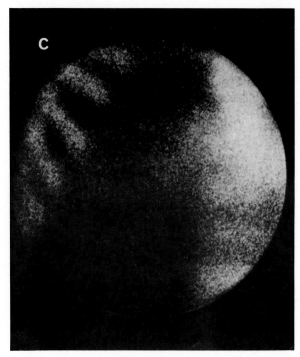

Figure 8, continued.

not be misinterpreted as recurrent neoplastic disease (8). Radiation sialadenitis commonly occurs in the first 6 months after radiation therapy, but salivary gland uptake may persist for years after treatment. It has been observed in other diseases that also affect salivary gland function, such as lupus erythematosus, renal failure, and Sjogren's syndrome.

Faint to moderate salivary gland uptake may occasionally occur in patients who have not received cervical irradiation and have no disease that affects the salivary glands.

Lung Uptake

Pulmonary activity of moderate intensity not associated with obvious pulmonary pathology is occasionally seen on 6- and 24-hour images and subsequently fades on later views. Prominent lung uptake may also be seen in scans performed after lymphography (7), as shown in Figure 11. Therefore, if lymphography and ^{67}Ga scans are planned as part of a tumor staging evaluation, it is preferable to perform the ^{67}Ga scan prior to the lymphogram.

Splenic Uptake

Uptake in the spleen is highly variable, even in the absence of direct splenic involvement with tumor or infection. Most scans demonstrate some splenic up-

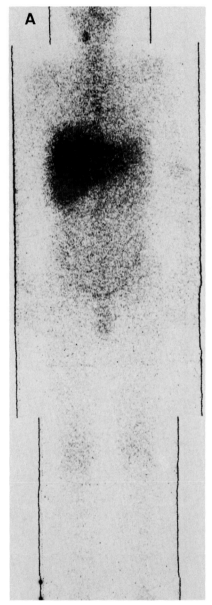

Figure 9. Gallium scan (A) demonstrates a cervical node, but the liver is apparently normal. A liver scan, obtained immediately prior to administration of ^{67}Ga citrate, demonstrates a large lesion in the right lobe of the liver, as seen on the anterior view (B), in this patient with a hepatoma. When a hepatic lesion is suspected, the ^{67}Ga scan cannot be interpreted without a ^{99m}Tc-sulfur colloid scan, because uptake in lesion and liver is often equal, resulting in apparently "normal" liver uptake.

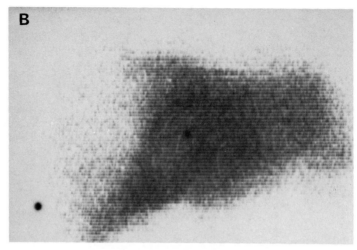

Figure 9, continued.

take, and most causes of splenomegaly are associated with increased uptake. In patients with Hodgkin's disease, it is not uncommon to observe splenomegaly and increased ^{67}Ga uptake in the spleen and yet find no evidence of splenic tumor at staging laparotomy. An example is shown in Figure 12.

NORMAL PEDIATRIC ^{67}Ga SCAN

The pattern of normal ^{67}Ga uptake in the child is somewhat different from that in adults. Bowel activity is seen less frequently, and the abdomen is therefore easier to evaluate. Activity is seen in the epiphyseal regions and may be seen in the thymus. It is not known if epiphyseal uptake occurs in the bone matrix, the cartilagenous structures, or in the adjacent marrow. The uptake is most marked in the regions of most active bone growth. An example is shown in Figure 13.

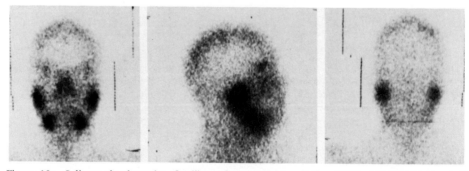

Figure 10.   Salivary gland uptake of gallium after cervical irradiation (4000 rads) for treatment of Hodgkin's disease seen in anterior, lateral, and posterior views. It is important not to confuse this uptake with recurrent tumor.

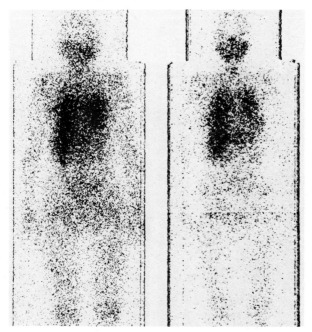

Figure 11. Pulmonary uptake in a patient who had prior lymphography. The oily contrast medium used in lymphography is partially trapped in the pulmonary circulation and may produce a local vascular reaction. This patient had a normal chest radiograph.

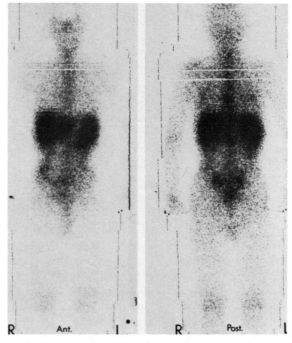

Figure 12. Increased splenic uptake of ^{67}Ga in a patient with Hodgkin's disease. Although the spleen was enlarged, no tumor was detected in the splenic parenchyma when sectioned. Increased splenic uptake in "reactive splenomegaly" and difficulty in detecting para-aortic and mesenteric lymph node involvement are two limitations in the use of ^{67}Ga for staging of Hodgkin's disease.

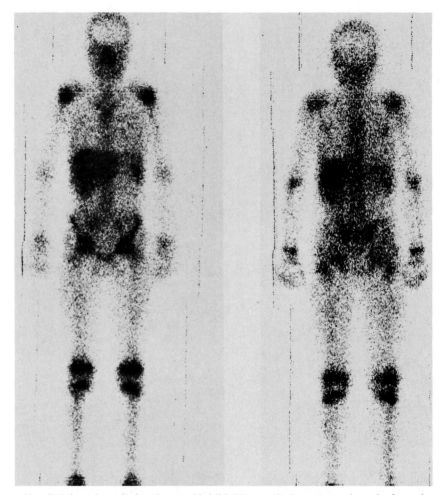

Figure 13.   Epiphyseal uptake in a 9-year-old child. The uptake is most prominent in the regions of major bone growth. This pattern of periarticular uptake may also be seen in young adults. (Courtesy of Dr. Carlos Bekerman.)

Thymic uptake in children often presents a clinical dilemma. Frequently, the ^{67}Ga scan is ordered to exclude neoplasm in a child with a "mediastinal mass" seen on chest x-ray. The pattern of ^{67}Ga uptake in the thymus is highly variable. Uptake may or may not be seen in a radiographically enlarged thymus gland. Conversely, thymic uptake can be observed in the absence of radiographically demonstrable enlargement, as seen in Figure 14. Most of the current information concerning ^{67}Ga uptake in the thymus is anecdotal; no large-scale evaluation of mediastinal uptake in children has been reported. Based on our observations, we do not recommend use of ^{67}Ga scanning for local evaluation of mediastinal masses in children. This procedure often produces information that only further complicates the diagnostic evaluation.

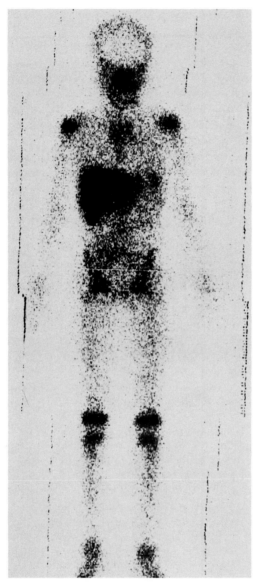

Figure 14. The thymus may be very prominent on gallium scans in children. It should not be misinterpreted as a neoplastic lesion. This 8-year-old girl had no evidence of disease in the mediastinum. (Courtesy of Dr. Carlos Bekerman.)

SUMMARY

The normal gallium image (8–11) has a characteristic appearance based on the biodistribution of ^{67}Ga citrate. However, there are many important variations in the normal pattern. These variations may appear in the absence of disease, under the influence of a variety of clinical situations. In addition, neoplastic and inflammatory lesions may cause gallium uptake that closely resembles normal patterns.

The appearance of the normal gallium image is strongly dependent on the time between injection of the radiopharmaceutical and performance of the study. For this reason, it is desirable that the procedure in each laboratory be standardized as much as possible with respect to the time between injected dose and image performance, views obtained, and format of data presentation. Attention to these details will enable the interpreting physician to more reliably assess the normal variation in ^{67}Ga imaging.

When there is uncertainty about the significance of a focus of activity, ancillary views, particularly lateral views, will frequently help separate normal structures from possible underlying pathology. Ancillary studies, such as the use of the ^{99m}Tc-sulfur colloid liver scan or orally administered ^{99m}Tc-sulfur colloid, may also be of help in differentiating physiologic from pathologic ^{67}Ga localization.

REFERENCES

1. Hartman RE, Hayes RL: The binding of gallium and indium by blood serum proteins, in 1967 Research Report, Medical Division, Oak Ridge Associated Universities, ORAU-106, Oak Ridge, Tenn., 1967.

2. Edwards CL, Hayes RL, Nelson B, et al: Radioactive gallium uptake in tumors, in 1969 Research Report, Medical Division, Oak Ridge Associated Universities, ORAU-110, Oak Ridge, Tenn., 1969.

3. Nelson B, Hayes RL, Edwards CL, et al: Distribution of gallium in human tissues after intravenous administration. *J Nucl Med* **13**:92, 1972.

4. Mishkin FS, Maynard WP: Lacrimal gland accumulation of ^{67}Ga. *J Nucl Med* **15**: 630, 1975.

5. Larson SM, Schall GL: Gallium-67 concentration in human breast milk. *J Amer Med Ass* **218**:257, 1971.

6. Bekerman C, Hoffer PB: Salivary gland uptake of ^{67}Ga-citrate following radiation therapy. *J Nucl Med* **17**:685, 1976.

7. Lentle BC, Castor WR, Khaliq A, et al: The effect of contrast lymphangiography on localization of ^{67}Ga citrate. *J Nucl Med* **16**:374, 1975.

8. Small RL, Bennett LR: Normal ^{67}Ga scan. *J Nucl Med* **12**:394, 1971.

9. Edwards CL, Hayes RL, Nelson B: The "normal" ^{67}Ga photoscan. *J Nucl Med* **13**:428, 1972.

10. Larson SM, Milder MS, Johnston GS: Interpretation of ^{67}Ga photoscan. *J Nucl Med* **14**:208, 1973.

11. Tedesco FJ, Coleman RE, Siegel BA: Gallium citrate (^{67}Ga) accumulation in pseudo-membranous colitis. *J Amer Med Ass,* **235**:59, 1976.

Part 2

The Use of Gallium in Diagnosing Inflammatory Disease

The initial use of gallium-67 was for detection and staging of malignancies. Occasionally, however, an area of increased uptake would be identified on scan that would subsequently prove to be due to inflammation rather than tumor.

These "false-positive" tumor scans were first believed to represent a deficiency of gallium scanning. Only slowly did the realization emerge that gallium scanning might also be useful as a method of detection of occult inflammatory disease.

The use of gallium scanning for detection of inflammatory lesions requires modification of the techniques usually used for tumor imaging. Speed is often critical. Also, it is important to understand the interrelation of the use of gallium with other methods of diagnosis, including conventional radiologic techniques, ultrasonography, and computed tomography. Finally, it is necessary to understand the pathologic anatomy of inflammatory lesions, especially the abdomen, where it is often difficult to detect and localize such lesions.

This section, therefore, contains a comprehensive discussion of the pathology and anatomy of the abdomen as it relates to inflammatory disease as well as a description of nonnuclear imaging techniques.

4

Anatomy and Pathology
of Intra-Abdominal Abscesses

Robert J. Churchill, M.D.

Assistant Clinical Professor of Radiology
Foster G. McGaw Hospital
Loyola University Medical Center
Maywood, Illinois

Carlos J. Reynes, M.D.

Director of Ultrasound and Whole Body
Computed Tomography
Associate Professor of Radiology
Foster G. McGaw Hospital
Loyola University Medical Center
Maywood, Illinois

Robert E. Henkin, M.D.

Director of Nuclear Medicine
Assistant Professor of Radiology
Foster G. McGaw Hospital
Loyola University Medical Center
Maywood, Illinois

PATHOLOGY OF INTRA-ABDOMINAL ABSCESSES

Intra-abdominal abscess formation remains an important and often perplexing clinical diagnostic problem. About 0.5% of patients undergoing elective abdominal surgery develop a subphrenic abscess (1,2). [About 85% of all subphrenic abscesses develop after elective or emergency abdominal surgical procedures (3,4).] The overall mortality rate of subphrenic abscesses ranges from 14 to 50% (3–11). If left untreated, the mortality rate can run as high as 94% (10). Proper drainage and appropriate antibiotic therapy remain the treatment of choice.

Approximately 20% of patients with subphrenic abscesses have multiple abscesses (3,9). Forty-nine percent of the patients in one study had residual, recurrent, or additional undrained abscesses; the mortality rate in this group of patients was more than two times higher than in the group that had adequate drainage initially (3). Early, aggressive, and accurate diagnostic intervention is therefore indicated so that the proper drainage route can be intelligently selected. To accomplish this goal, it is fundamental that one be cognizant not only of the predisposing factors in the patient's history but also of the intra- and extraperitoneal anatomy and dynamics involved in the spread and localization of inflammatory processes.

In an attempt to be complete, abdominal abscess in this chapter will be defined as "any collection of pus residing in the intraperitoneal or retroperitoneal space in either the abdomen or pelvis."

INTRAPERITONEAL ANATOMY

The peritoneal cavity can be divided into three major areas: the supramesocolic space, the inframesocolic space, and the pelvic cavity (12–15).

The supramesocolic space is the area located beneath the diaphragm and above the transverse mesocolon (Figure 1). This large space can be divided into four intraperitoneal spaces and one extraperitoneal space. Even though only two of these spaces are actually subphrenic (subdiaphragmatic), this whole area is collectively referred to as the subphrenic space. This terminology is anatomically incorrect, but because of common usage, supramesocolic and subphrenic remain synonymous terms.

The supramesocolic space is divided into right and left spaces by the falciform ligament superiorly and by the falciform ligament, ligamentum teres hepatis, and descending duodenum inferiorly. The right lobe of the liver is suspended by the coronary ligament from the posterior abdominal wall at the level of the posterior costophrenic sulcus (not from the dome of the diaphragm), thus creating a superior suprahepatic (subdiaphragmatic) space and an inferior subhepatic space on the right side (Figure 2a). These two spaces are sometimes divided by inflammatory membranes into anterior and posterior spaces (Figure 2b). The posterior inferior subhepatic space (hepatorenal fossa) is sometimes referred to as Morrison's pouch and lies between the kidney and right lobe of the liver. The third space on the right is extraperitoneal and lies between the leaves of the coronary ligament (bare area of the liver; Figure 2b). The right paracolic gutter is in communication with the subhepatic space on the right side.

Because the left lobe of the liver is small, the left suprahepatic and subhepatic spaces are generally continuous; this large space is referred to as the combined

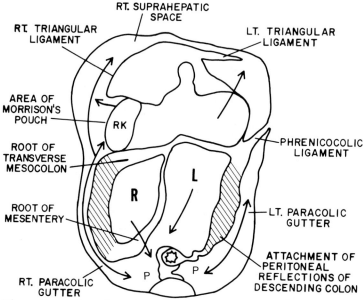

Figure 1.   The various peritoneal attachments and ligaments that partition the peritoneal cavity are shown on this anterior view. The supramesocolic space encompasses the entire region from the transverse mesocolon to the diaphragm and includes both the suprahepatic space and Morrison's pouch. The right (R) and left (L) infracolic spaces are divisions of the inframesocolic space that are situated below the transverse mesocolon and above the pelvic cavity (P). Arrows indicate the major pathways of flow of free fluid; RK, right kidney. [Redrawn from Meyers (14).]

left subphrenic space (9). The second space on the left is posterior to the stomach and is the lesser sac (Figure 3). The left paracolic gutter is not in communication with the combined subphrenic space because of the barrier produced by the phrenicocolic ligament (14,16) (Figure 1).

The inframesocolic space is located below the transverse mesocolon and above the pelvic brim. Laterally located are the right and left paracolic gutters. Medial to the ascending and descending colons are the infracolic spaces. The right infracolic space is bounded by the ascending colon, transverse mesocolon, and root of the small bowel mesentery. The larger left infracolic space is bounded by the transverse mesocolon and descending colon but is freely open inferiorly to the pelvic cavity (14) (Figure 1).

The pelvic cavity lies below the pelvic brim. It contains a central cul-de-sac (pouch of Douglas) and paravesical recesses on each side of the bladder. The paracolic gutters and left infracolic space freely communicate with the pelvic cavity.

DYNAMICS OF FLUID FLOW

Autio (17) and Meyers (12–14) detailed the method of spread of intraperitoneal fluid by instilling positive contrast material into the peritoneal cavity. Meyers (14) has demonstrated that multiple factors influence the flow of free fluid in the peritoneal cavity that contribute to the eventual areas of localization. Among these factors are the originating site and rate of outpouring of fluid, the characteristics of the fluid, gravity, intra-abdominal pressure gradients, body habitus,

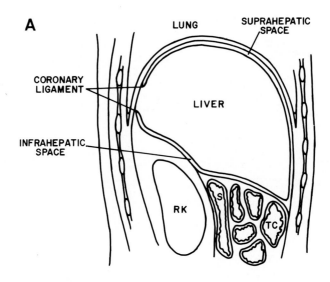

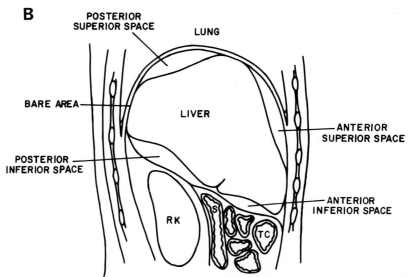

Figure 2.   Longitudinal section. The right supramesocolic space is divided into a superior suprahepatic space and an inferior subhepatic space by the coronary ligament (A). The bare area (B) is a third space (extraperitoneal) that lies between the leaves of the coronary ligament. Abscesses may be compartmentalized into anterior and posterior spaces (B) by adhesions. RK, right kidney; S, stomach; TC, transverse colon.

mesenteric reflections and attachments, and peritoneal recesses. The lowest gravitational area in the upright or supine patient is the pelvis. The area of lowest pressure, due primarily to respiratory motion, is the subphrenic space.

The usual route of fluid flow in the peritoneal cavity is into the pelvis up the paracolic gutters (primarily on the right) and into the right subhepatic space (12–14,17). While fliud may move from the right subhepatic space to the right suprahepatic space, the predominant collection area is the subhepatic space. The

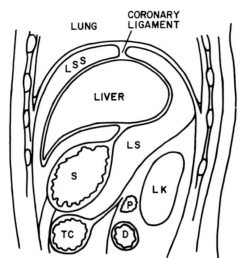

Figure 3.   Longitudinal section. The left supramesocolic space consists of two major spaces: the combined subphrenic space (LSS) and the lesser sac (LS). LK, left kidney; D, duodenum; P pancreas; S, stomach; TC, transverse colon. [Redrawn from Meyers (14).]

phrenicocolic ligament acts as a natural barrier to flow into the subphrenic space on the left side (14). Fluid placed in the right subhepatic space may also reach the pelvis and left paracolic gutter (Figure 1). These dynamics occur in both recumbant and upright positions. Because of these flow patterns, inflammatory fluid that is not walled off early can produce abscesses far removed from the initial site of contamination.

The experimental findings of Autio and Meyers correlate fairly well with the usual location of intra-abdominal abscesses. Harley reported that 65% of intraperitoneal abscesses occur near the initial inflammatory event, while 32% seemed to be the result of generalized peritonitis or spread from a distant site (18). The majority of subphrenic abscesses occur on the right side, and most of them are in the right subhepatic space (9,14). These abscesses can occur following leaks from a perforated viscus anywhere in the abdomen, from regional inflammatory processes, liver and biliary tract surgery, gastric surgery, and generalized peritonitis. Left subphrenic abscesses, on the other hand, more commonly occur after perforated gastric ulcers, regional anastomotic leaks, gastrectomy, and splenectomy. A high incidence of left subphrenic abscess formation has been noted when both gastrectomy and splenectomy have been performed concomitantly (3).

Lesser sac abscesses rarely result from the spread of an inflammatory process through the foramen of Winslow (14,15,17). The majority of lesser sac abscesses occur secondary to a regional process, such as perforated ulcer or pancreatitis. Pelvic abscesses can develop after peritonitis, anastomotic leaks, diverticulitis, and pelvic inflammatory disease.

While the majority of inflammatory processes are walled off before generalized spread can occur, a significant number are not. Therefore, when intra-abdominal abscess is suspected, the entire abdomen should be carefully searched, regardless of the location of the suspected source.

RETROPERITONEAL ANATOMY

As many as 40% of all intra-abdominal abscesses involve the retroperitoneal space (19). The retroperitoneal space is bounded anteriorly by the posterior parietal peritoneum and posteriorly by the transversalis fascia (Figure 4). The anatomy of this region has been superbly described by Meyers (14,20)

The space immediately posterior to the posterior parietal peritoneum and anterior to the anterior renal fascia is the anterior pararenal space; it contains the pancreas, duodenal sweep, ascending and descending colon, and retroperitoneal appendix (Figure 4). There is a potential communication across the midline of this space at the level of the pancreas. The anterior pararenal space is limited laterally by the lateroconal fascia. Inflammatory processes in this space can extend medially across the lateral psoas margin as far as the midline; however, the psoas margin is not obliterated. Lateral extension does not destroy the properitoneal fat line (flank stripe) (14,20).

The perirenal space is bounded by the renal (Gerota's) fascia and contains the kidneys, adrenals, and perirenal fat. Medially, this space is bounded by the psoas muscle fascia and connective tissue at the level of the aorta and inferior vena cava. Laterally, it forms the lateroconal fascia, which fuses with the peritoneal reflection, forming the paracolic gutters (Figure 4). The psoas margin at the level of the kidney and the renal outline can be obliterated by an inflammatory process in this space; however, the properitoneal fat line is preserved (14,20).

The posterior pararenal space is bounded anteriorly by the posterior renal fascia and posteriorly by the transversalis fascia. It contains only fat and continues laterally as the properitoneal fat line. Medially, it follows the psoas margin (Figure 4). Inflammatory processes in this space obliterate the properitoneal fat line and the inferior psoas margin. All three spaces have a potential communication at the level of the iliac fossa (14,20).

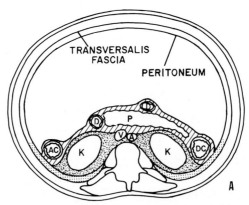

Figure 4.   Transverse (A) and longitudinal (B) sections that show the three retroperitoneal spaces. The lined area is the anterior pararenal space, the densely speckled area is the pararenal space, and the dotted area is the posterior pararenal space. A detailed cross-sectional drawing (C) shows the fascias that divide the various spaces. The transverse sections are viewed, according to convention, with the patient's right on the viewer's left. A, aorta; AC, ascending colon; D, duodenum; DC, descending colon; K, kidney; P, pancreas; PM, psoas muscle; V, inferior vena cava. [Redrawn from Meyers (20).]

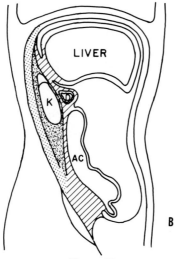

Figure 4B.

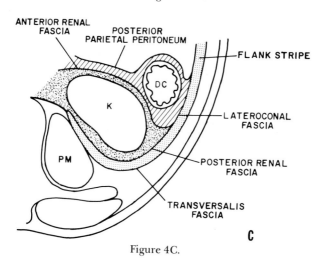

Figure 4C.

Once a general knowledge of the anatomy and patterns of fluid flow within the abdomen is achieved, search for occult inflammatory lesions can proceed on a more logical basis.

REFERENCES

1. Halliday P, Lowenthal J: Subphrenic abscess. *Austral New Zeal J Surg* **33**:360, 1964.
2. Sanders RC: The changing epidemiology of subphrenic abscess and its clinical and radiological consequences. *Brit J Surg* **57**:449, 1970.
3. DeCross JJ, Poulin TL, Fos PS, et al: Subphrenic abscess. *Surg Gynecol Obstet* **138**(6):841, 1974.
4. Sherman JJ, Davis JR, Jesseph JE: Subphrenic abscess; a continuing hazard. *Amer J Surg* **117**:117, 1969.

5. Bonfils-Roberts EA, Barone JE, Nealon TF: Treatment of subphrenic abscess. *Surg Clin N Amer* **55**(6):1361, 1975.

6. Carter RN, Brewer IA: Subphrenic abscess, a thoraco-abdominal clinical complex. *Amer J Surg* **108**:165, 1964.

7. DePalma AE: The subphrenic abscess: a clinical review. *J Med Soc New Jersey* **66**:250, 1969.

8. Halasz NA: Subphrenic abscess: myths and facts. *J Amer Med Ass* **214**:724, 1970.

9. Konvolinka CW, Olearczyk A: Subphrenic abscess. *Current Problems Surg,* Jan. 1972.

10. Magilligan DJ: Suprahepatic abscess. *Amer J Surg* **86**:14, 1968.

11. Smith EB: Subphrenic abscess: a surgical enigma. *J Nat Med Ass* **68**(1):55, 1976.

12. Meyers MA: The spread and localization of acute intraperitoneal effusions. *Radiology* **95**:547, 1970.

13. Meyers MA: Peritoneography: normal and pathologic anatomy. *Amer J Roentgenol Radium Ther Nucl Med* **117**:353, 1973.

14. Meyers MA: Dynamic Radiology of the Abdomen: Normal and Pathologic Anatomy, New York, Springer-Verlag, 1976, pp. 1–35, 113–194.

15. Sanders RC: Radiological and radioisotopic diagnosis of perihepatic abscess. *CRC Crit Rev Clin Radiol Nucl Med* **5**:165, 1974.

16. Meyers MA: Roentgen significance of the phrenicocolic ligament. *Radiology* **95**:539, 1970.

17. Autio V: The spread of intraperitoneal infection. Studies with roentgen contrast media. *Acta Chir Scand Suppl* **321**:1, 1964.

18. Harley HRS: Subphrenic Abscess, Springfield, Ill., Charles C Thomas, 1955, p. 112.

19. Altemeier WA, Culbertson WR, Fullen WD, et al: Intra-abdominal abscesses. *Amer J Surg* **125**:70, 1973.

20. Meyers MA: Acute extraperitoneal infection. *Sem Roentgenol* **8**:445, 1973.

5

Radiographic and Ultrasonic Methods of Diagnosing Intra-Abdominal Abscesses

Robert J. Churchill, M.D.

Assistant Clinical Professor of Radiology
Foster G. McGaw Hospital
Loyola University Medical Center
Maywood, Illinois

Carlos J. Reynes, M.D.

Director of Ultrasound and Whole Body
Computed Tomography
Associate Professor of Radiology
Foster G. McGaw Hospital
Loyola University Medical Center
Maywood, Illinois

Until relatively recently, the only anatomic methods of localizing intra-abdominal abscesses were physical examination and a variety of radiographic procedures. While the advent of gallium scanning has added a new dimension to the diagnosis of abscesses, it is still important to have a general understanding of the radiographic procedures that are useful. It is also important to appreciate the value and limitations of two new imaging modalities, ultrasound and whole-body computed tomography.

RADIOGRAPHIC EXAMINATIONS

Plain-film Studies

Preliminary plain x-ray films, which consist of an upright postero-anterior chest, supine and upright abdomen, and a left lateral decubitus (right side up) abdomen film, are routine in a evaluation of a suspected intra-abdominal abscess. The only pathognomonic sign of an abscess is a collection of gas that appears to be extraintestinal and remains in the same location despite patient positional change. This finding has been reported to occur in 30–61% of patients with subphrenic abscesses (1–8). Extraluminal gas in a febrile patient almost certainly indicates an abscess. Rarely, a loculated pneumoperitoneum may occur in a postsurgical patient and could result in a false-positive diagnosis. Also, hemorrhage into the gastrointestinal tract or retroperitoneal space (e.g., leaking aortic aneurysm) can produce mottled radiolucencies on radiographics that mimic the pattern of abscess gas (9,10).

Knowledge of the intraperitoneal and retroperitoneal anatomy often enables one to determine the anatomic space the abscess occupies (Figure 1). Because inflammatory membranes usually compartmentalize abscesses, gas shadows seen in the frontal plane can actually be in one of several spaces. Multiple views, including a cross-table lateral, are often helpful for anatomic localization.

Intra-abdominal abscesses commonly contain an air-fluid level that is seen on dependent views of the abdomen (Figure 2). Pelvic abscesses often present also with a superimposed small bowel obstruction due to a loop of small bowel being entrapped in the inflammatory process (Figure 3). We have seen this finding several times with perforated diverticulitis and perforation due to a foreign body. Air-fluid levels in an abscess in the left upper quadrant must be differentiated from an air-fluid level in the stomach (Figure 4).

Other plain-film findings include a soft-tissue mass (1–48%) (2,5,11) (Figure 5); organ displacement; fixation of a mobile organ; obliteration of structures normally seen, such as psoas margin, renal outline, or flank stripe (Figure 6); pleural effusion (42–89%) (1,2,3,5,7,8,11); elevation of the diaphragm (33–95%) (1,2,3,5,7,8,11); scoliosis; atelectasis (70–75%) (1,3,5); and adynamic ileus (59%) (3). It is often difficult to decide how much emphasis to place on any single finding in a recently postoperative patient who may have any number of noninflammatory problems, such as basilar atelectasis, pulmonary infarction, or reflex ileus; however, a combination of radiologic findings is highly suggestive of abscess.

Carter and Brewer refer to the thoracoabdominal complex in subphrenic abscess (4). Eighty-six percent of the patients in their study had both thoracic

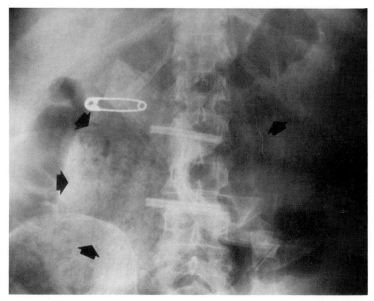

Figure 1. Supine radiograph that demonstrates a pattern of mottled radiolucencies (arrows) that crosses the midline and conforms to the anatomic area of the pancreas. Both the increased space between stomach and transverse colon and the inflammatory changes along the greater curvature of the stomach are further evidence that this postoperative abscess is located in the pancreas and lesser sac.

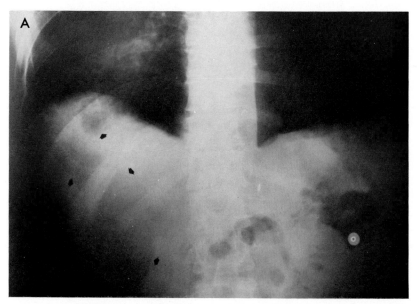

Figure 2. A supine radiograph (A) shows an elevated right hemidiaphragm and two gas collections in the right upper quadrant (arrows). A left lateral decubitus film (B) demonstrates an air fluid level in each of the two gas collections. The abscesses were in the anterior and posterior suprahepatic spaces.

51

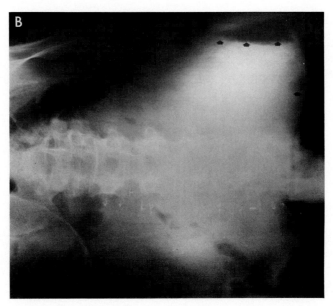

Figure 2, continued.

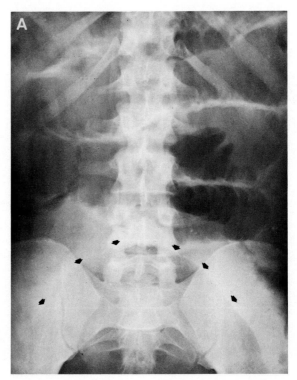

Figure 3.　A supine radiograph (A) shows a mechanical bowel obstruction and a large radiolucent structure (arrows) in the projection of the pelvis. An air fluid level (arrows) in a large pelvic abscess is seen on the left lateral decubitus film (B). (Courtesy of Dr. Leon Love, Loyola University Medical Center, Maywood, Illinois.)

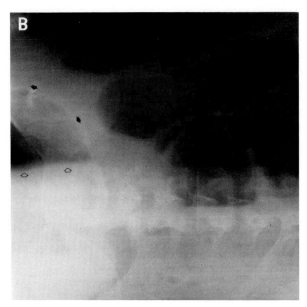

Figure 3, continued.

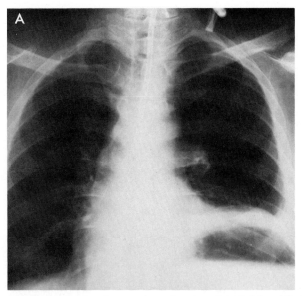

Figure 4.   An upright chest x-ray (A) demonstrates elevation of the left hemidiaphragm and a left pleural effusion. The large structure that contains an air fluid level could represent the gastric fundus or an abscess. The increased space between this structure and the diaphragm may be due to a subpulmonic collection of fluid. After a barium meal, the right lateral decubitus film (B) shows the abscess with an air fluid level separate from the stomach. Note also the extrinsic pressure on the splenic flexure. (Courtesy of Dr. Leon Love, Loyola University Medical Center, Maywood, Illinois.)

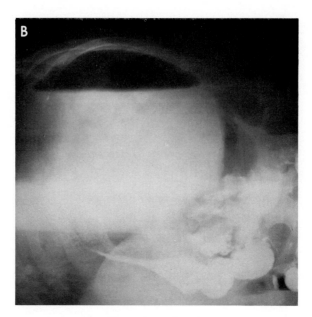

Figure 4, continued.

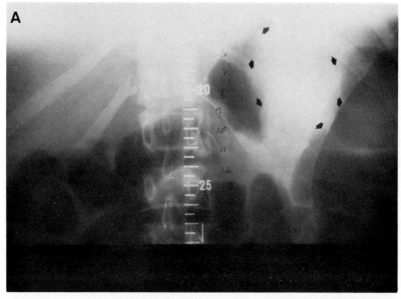

Figure 5A. Preliminary scanogram film taken prior to computed tomographic whole-body scanning in a patient who had become febrile after endoscopic retrograde pancreatography demonstrates a left upper quadrant, soft-tissue density mass (arrows) that displaces the gastric and splenic flexure gas shadows.

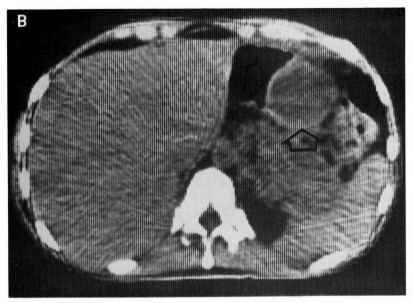

Figure 5B.   Computed tomographic scan (patient's right is on viewer's left) taken at the 18 cm mark shows an encapsulated mass that corresponds to the mass seen on the preliminary film. The density of the mass measured intermediate between water and liver density and was interpreted as an abscess, probably an infected pancreatic pseudocyst.

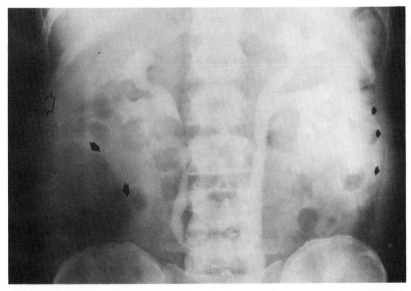

Figure 6.   Supine film from an intravenous pyelogram series demonstrates a gas-containing abcess (large closed arrows) in the right paracolic gutter. The inflammatory process has invaded the abdominal wall and obliterates a portion of the properitoneal fat line (open arrows). The normal left properitoneal flank stripe (small closed arrows) is visualized. (Courtesy of Dr. Leon Love, Loyola University Medical Center, Maywood, Illinois.)

55

and abdominal findings, with 44% having predominantly thoracic changes and 42% having predominantly abdominal findings. The most common thoracic findings are basilar infiltrates or atelectasis, pleural effusion, and an elevated diaphragm. Whenever pleural effusion is suspected, a lateral decubitus chest film should be performed. This procedure will allow detection of a subpulmonic collection of fluid that may be the cause of a seemingly elevated diaphragm. It is important to know whether a combined liver-lung isotope scan is to be performed, because a subpulmonic pleural effusion may result in a false-positive interpretation of suprahepatic abscess.

Fluoroscopy

Fluoroscopy of the diaphragm can be used to detect total or localized restricted motion. This finding has been reported to occur in 25–100% of patients with subphrenic abscess (1–5,7,8,11). It occurs more often with suprahepatic abscesses and left-sided abscesses (5). A preferable method of evaluation of diaphragmatic motion is by ultrasound examination.

Contrast Studies

Positive contrast examinations of the gastrointestinal tract are helpful in determining if gas collections are extraluminal. Barium is the medium of choice, unless an anastomotic leak or perforation is suspected, in which case one of the water-soluble contrast agents should be used. These procedures are utilized mostly to evaluate gas collections in the left upper quadrant, where stomach, small bowel, and colon gas can cause the most confusion (Figure 7).

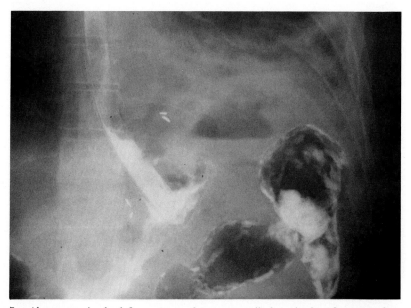

Figure 7.   Abscess gas in the left upper quadrant can easily be mistaken for stomach or colon. Administration of contrast medium in this case delineates the stomach and colon and establishes the gas as extraluminal. (Courtesy of Dr. Richard Cooper, Loyola University Medical Center, Maywood, Illinois.)

Before ultrasonography was available, double-contrast peritoneography was occasionally used to delineate the various peritoneal recesses and organ surfaces. This method was useful in establishing the patency of communication of the various peritoneal recesses. The method, however, cannot distinguish between obliteration due to recent abscess and that due to fibrosis from an older lesion or surgery.

Intravenous excretory urography may be employed for evaluation of perirenal, renal, and other retroperitoneal regions (Figure 8). Right ureteral obstruction at the level of the pelvic brim may be seen with periappendiceal or tube-ovarian abscesses, but ureteral calculi, terminal ileitis, and leukemic ileocecal syndrome cause identical changes.

Another occasionally useful procedure is infusion tomography (12). A routine drip infusion used for excretory urography is performed and then followed by tomography of the organ or area suspected of containing an abscess. Use of this technique has been reported for liver abscesses (13,14) (Figure 9). The hepatic abscess is observed as a radiolucent area surrounded by a contrast enhanced rim.

Arteriography has been employed for both hepatic and subphrenic abscesses. Subphrenic abscess collections result in displacement of the main hepatic vessels and medial displacement of the lateral liver edge (15). Intrahepatic abscesses displace the intrahepatic vessels (Figure 10). These abscesses may be hypovascular or vascular, and a hypervascular rim may be seen. Sometimes the distinction between intra- and extrahepatic abscesses cannot be made with certainty (16).

Draining sinus tracts may be injected with a water-soluble contrast material to delineate the size and position of an abscess cavity (Figure 11). With this procedure, as with all other radiographic procedures, multiple views, including a

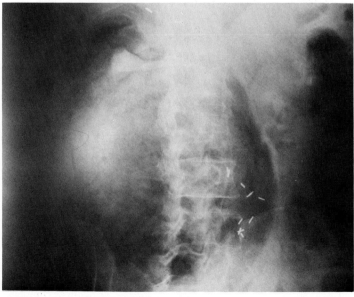

Figure 8.   A left posterior oblique projection of an intravenous pyelogram demonstrates displacement of the right kidney by a gas-producing infection (*Clostridia*) that began in a large simple renal cyst in a nondiabetic patient.

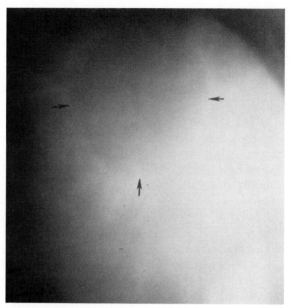

Figure 9.   Tomogram of the liver after contrast infusion in the right posterior oblique position demonstrates a radiolucent mass (hypovascular) with a peripheral hypervascular rim (arrows) in a patient with a positive indirect hemagglutination (IHA) reaction for *Entamoeba histolytica.* [From Morin et al. (14). By permission of *Journal of the American Medical Association.*]

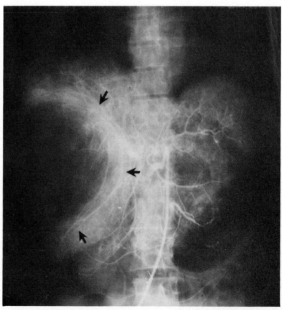

Figure 10.   Arteriogram of an intrahepatic abscess (amebic) demonstrates displacement of the vessels by a hypovascular mass. The area surrounding the abscess is hypervascular. (Courtesy of Dr. J. M. Cardoso, Mexico City, Mexico.)

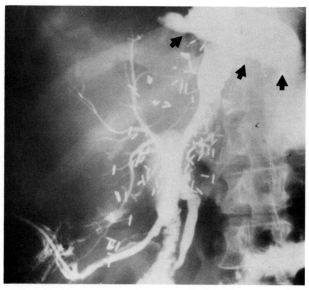

Figure 11.   A T-tube cholangiogram shows a large collection of contrast material in the epigastric area (arrows). Purulent material drained from the T tube after the study, but the fever persisted. An abscess was found in this area at laparotomy.

lateral view, are needed for accurate localization. Follow-up studies are valuable for documentation of the decrease in size of a draining cavity.

ULTRASOUND

Diagnostic ultrasound is now employed routinely in the evaluation of patients with suspected abscesses. This procedure should be performed after appropriate plain-film examinations have been obtained; correlation with a gallium scan is almost always recommended.

The diagnostic accuracy of ultrasound in detecting intra-abdominal abscesses is reported as 86–95% (17,18). The sonographic pattern of an abscess may vary from a totally sonolucent, cystic mass (Figure 12) to one that appears to be entirely solid. Most commonly, masses with mixed echo patterns are seen (Figure 13). The majority of abscesses are irregular in contour, have thick shaggy walls, and are predominantly cystic (Figure 14). Differentiation in the abdomen from other complex structures, such as hematoma (Figure 15), necrotic tumor, or phlegmon, and in the pelvis from endometriosis or ectopic pregnancy usually cannot be made on the echographic findings alone. The fluid-filled bowel generally has a tubular configuration and changes shape during the examination. If the distinction cannot be made, a repeat examination on the following day usually resolves the dilemma. A fluid-filled stomach can cause confusion. If there is any doubt, a nasogastric tube should be passed and the fluid aspirated.

Excessive bowel gas prevents an adequate examination. Therefore, patients should be prepared if possible with oral simethicone for 24–48 hours before the

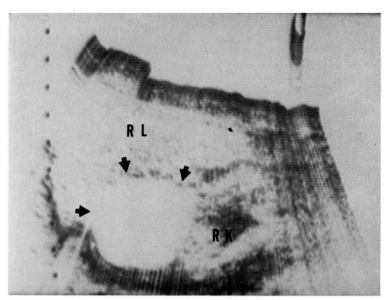

Figure 12. A febrile neonate with a history of traumatic delivery had an ultrasonogram (longitudinal scan 4 cm to the right of midline) that revealed a totally sonolucent mass cephlad to the right kidney (arrows). At surgery, the lesion proved to be an abscess associated with an adrenal hemorrhage. RL, right lobe of the liver; RK, right kidney.

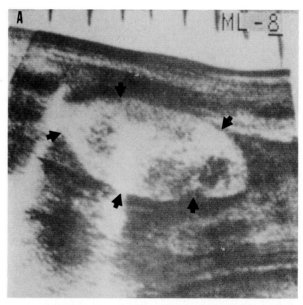

Figure 13. A 16-year-old male with a history of diarrhea and fever was suspected of having inflammatory bowel disease. An ultrasonogram demonstrated a mass adjacent to the left kidney of mixed density compatible with an inflammatory process or necrotic tumor (arrows). A chronic perirenal abscess of the left kidney was found at surgery. LK, left kidney; RK, right kidney.

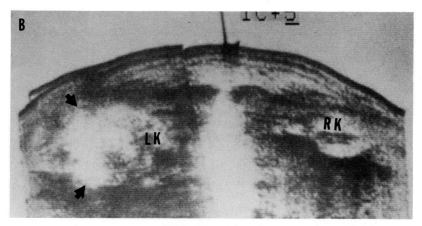

Figure 13, continued.

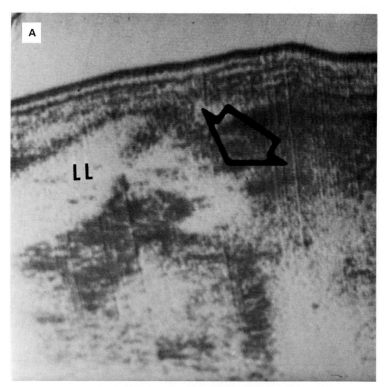

Figure 14.   Longitudinal (midline) and transverse (level of the pancreas) ultrasonograms show cystic structures with irregular walls and some internal echoes in a postsurgical patient. Multiple abscesses were found at surgery. LL, left lobe of the liver; RK, right kidney.

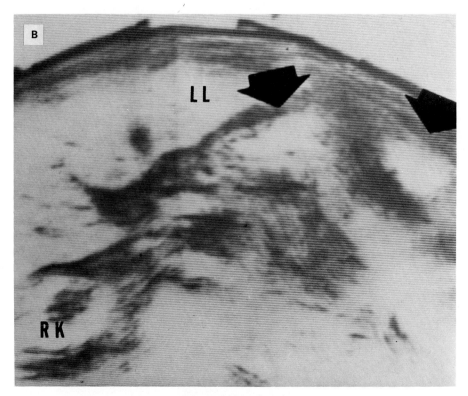

Figure 14, continued.

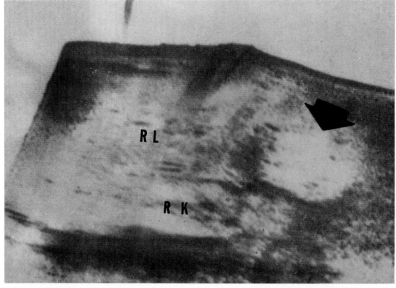

Figure 15. Longitudinal ultrasonogram (7 cm to the right of the midline) demonstrates a hematoma (arrow) in a postsurgical patient that is echographically identical to an abscess. RL, right lobe of the liver; RK, right kidney.

ultrasound examination. Bowel gas does not interfere with the ultrasonic evaluation of right subphrenic spaces. Both suprahepatic and subhepatic spaces are clearly seen, and distinction between subpulmonic and subphrenic collections of fluid is easily made. Diaphragmatic motion is routinely checked during the examination. The left subphrenic space is much more difficult to evaluate, particularly in patients who have had a splenectomy, because colon and stomach gas prevents sonic transmission.

The pelvis is an ideal location to search for abscess formation with ultrasound. The bladder must be distended to push the gas-containing bowel out of the pelvic cavity. This distended bladder, in addition, acts as a sonic window and a reference structure with which one can compare other cystic-appearing masses. Care must be taken not to overdistend the bladder, because it may push an abscess out of the pelvis into a region of gas-containing bowel.

Computed Tomographic Scanning

Computer-assisted tomographic (CT) whole-body scanning is a new imaging modality. Transverse, cross-sectional images are constructed by computer processing of several thousand informational points that represent linear x-ray attenuation coefficients that are taken during a scanning sequence. The resolution and image clarity permit identification of the normal anatomy and of pathologic processes (Figure 5). Enough experience has not yet been gained to determine if the density readings of abscesses are sufficiently specific to differentiate them from other solid or cystic lesions. A recent study did, however, detect 20 of 22 abscesses with CT scanning (19). The density readings ranged between 2 and 25 new Hounsfield units (NHU). It should be noted that pseudocysts, liver cysts, hematomas, endometriomas, and seromas had similar density readings. It must be reemphasized that pertinent historical data are needed for meaningful interpretation. The chief limitations of CT examination for abdominal abscess include the presence of barium and metallic surgical clips, excessive bowel gas motion with second-generation scanners, and the fact that abscesses may be equal in density to noninflammatory masses and fluid collections. In general, CT is most helpful in defining the exact anatomic extent of an abscess once its general location has been determined. The combined use of gallium scanning to detect and CT to define the lesion may prove to be a useful approach to evaluating abscesses.

SUMMARY

Conventional radiographic methods are extremely useful for detection of abdominal abscesses. They are usually rapidly performed and often exquisitely specific in localizing the region of involvement. The chief drawback of these methods is their limited sensitivity. The two newest imaging modalities, ultrasonography and computed tomography, provide excellent anatomic characterization of inflammatory lesions. Both methods are best utilized when some anatomic direction, either by signs and symptoms or by results of other diagnostic tests, is known to direct the examination to a specific region of the abdomen. Also, in a small number of patients, an adequate examination cannot always be obtained either because of artifacts from bowel gas, barium, and surgical clips or because of lack of patient cooperation.

Therefore, despite the value of these techniques, there is still need for a method of abscess detection that is very sensitive, regardless of the location of the lesion, and that can determine the general anatomic area of involvement. The gallium scan, to be discussed in the next chapter, is well suited for this task.

REFERENCES

1. DeCross JJ, Poulin TL, Fos PS, et al: Subphrenic abscess. *Surg Gynecol Obstet* **138**:841, 1974.

2. Sherman JJ, Davis JR, Jesseph JE; Subphrenic abscess; a continuing hazard. *Amer J Surg* **117**:117, 1969.

3. Bonfils-Roberts EA, Barone JE, Nealon TF: Treatment of subphrenic abscess. *Surg Clin N Amer* **55**:1361, 1975.

4. Carter RN, Brewer LA: Subphrenic abscess, a thoraco-abdominal clinical complex. *Amer J Surg* **108**:165, 1964.

5. Konvolinka CW, Olearczyk A: Subphrenic abscess. *Current Problems Surg,* Jan. 1972.

6. Altemeier WA, Culbertson WR, Fullen WD, et al: Intra-abdominal abscesses. *Amer J Surg* **125**:70, 1973.

7. Miller WT, Talman EA: Subphrenic abscess. *Amer J Roentgenol Radium Ther Nucl Med* **101**:961, 1967.

8. Wetterfors J: Subphrenic abscess: a clinical study of 101 cases. *Acta Chir Scand* **117**:388, 1959.

9. Nichols GB, Schilling PJ: Pseudo-retroperitoneal gas in rupture of aneurysm of abdominal aorta. *Amer J Roentgenol Radium Ther Nucl Med* **125**:134, 1975.

10. Han SY, Witten DM, Prim HS: Plain film diagnosis of massive gastrointestinal hemorrhage, in 76th Annual Meeting of the American Roentgen Ray Society, September 30 to October 3, 1975.

11. Magilligan DJ: Suprahepatic abscess. *Amer J Surg* **86**:14, 1968.

12. Rabushka S, Love L, Moncada R: Infusion tomography of the gallbladder. *Radiology* **109**:549, 1973.

13. Cardoso JM, Rodriguez J, Kimura K, et al: Detection of space occupying lesions of the liver by infusion tomography, in 61st Scientific Assembly, Radiological Society of North America, December 1975.

14. Morin ME, Baker DA, Marsan RE: Hepatic abscess: diagnosis in the adult by total body opacification. *J Amer Med Ass* **236**:1607, 1976.

15. Deutsch V, Adar R, Mozes M: Angiography in the diagnosis of subphrenic abscess. *Clin Radiol* **25**:133, 1974.

16. Reuter SR, Redman HC: Gastrointestinal Angiography, Philadelphia, Saunders, 1972, p. 196.

17. Jensen P, Pedersen JF: The value of ultrasonic scanning in the diagnosis of intra-abdominal abscesses and hematoma. *Surg Gynecol Obstet* **139**:326, 1974.

18. Doust BD: The use of ultrasound in the diagnosis of gastroenterological disease. *Gastroenterology* **70**:602, 1976.

19. Haaga JR, Alfidi RJ, Havrilla TR, et al: CT detection and aspiration of abdominal abscesses. *Amer J Roentgenol Radium Ther Nucl Med* **128**:465, 1977.

6

Gallium-67 in the Diagnosis of Inflammatory Disease

Robert E. Henkin, M.D.

Director of Nuclear Medicine
Assistant Professor of Radiology
Foster G. McGaw Hospital
Loyola University Medical Center
Maywood, Illinois

The traditional nuclear medicine techniques employed to localize intra-abdominal abscesses have been the liver-spleen scan and the combined liver-lung (either emission or transmission) scan to identify intrahepatic and subdiaphragmatic abscesses, respectively.

The finding of a single filling defect on a ^{99m}Tc-sulfur colloid liver scan is, unfortunately, nonspecific; the differential diagnosis includes abscess, cyst, benign tumor, malignant tumor, hemangioma, hematoma, and focal nodular hyperplasia. Multiple defects on a liver scan may also be seen with liver abscesses but also occur with metastatic disease, multiple hemangiomas, or polycystic disease. The combined liver-lung scan is also nonspecific when used to diagnose subphrenic abscesses. The separation between the liver and lung identified on such a scan may be due to any one of several etiologies, including subpulmonic effusion, inflammatory disease in the lung, or a serous fluid collection between the diaphragm and liver (1).

During the early period of clinical investigation of gallium-67 (^{67}Ga) citrate for tumor imaging, "false-positive" areas of gallium uptake were observed due to inflammatory lesions (2). Lavender and associates observed two such cases during a study undertaken to evaluate gallium scanning in a variety of neoplasms, one due to a breast abscess and the other due to a lung abscess. Lavender and colleagues made the astute observation that it would be useful to employ gallium for abscess imaging (3).

In 1972, Lomas and Wagner described the value of gallium scanning in the diagnosis of cholecystitis (4). In 1973, Littenberg and associates reported on a group of 12 patients, 11 of whom had focal inflammatory disease. All 11 were detected by the gallium scan (5). These reports provided the first documentation of the clinical value of gallium for searching out inflammatory disease.

Unlike liver-spleen or combined liver-lung imaging techniques, gallium imaging for abscesses is not restricted to any one organ or region. The former techniques depend on organ or tissue displacement, that is, indirect effects, and therefore have only a 60% sensitivity for detection of *perihepatic* (versus 70–85% for intrahepatic) inflammatory disease. (6). Gallium is a direct scanning agent with sensitivity for abscess detection in the 90% range.

TECHNICAL CONSIDERATIONS

The general technical considerations of gallium scanning are outlined in Chapter 2. However, imaging of inflammatory lesions often requires special modifications in technique. Patients undergoing scanning to localize inflammatory process are often acutely ill. The standard 72-hour delay for a gallium scan is, therefore, frequently undesirable. In addition, the vast majority of patients with suspected intra-abdominal abscess have had recent surgery. In many of these patients, vigorous bowel cleansing is contraindicated.

Early investigations of gallium uptake in inflammatory lesions revealed that the standard 72-hour delay was usually unnecessary (3). One comparison of early and delayed gallium scintigraphy in a small series of patients with potential subphrenic abscesses revealed that patients who had positive 6-hour scans also had positive 24- and 48-hour scans (7). Moreover, no patient whose scan was negative at 6 hours had a later positive scan. This observation does not conform precisely with our experience. We have studied two patients who had normal scans at 6 hours but who had demonstrable lesions at 24 hours. Both of the infections were due to anaerobic organisms. Therefore, while 48- and 72-hour delayed scans are often neither desirable nor possible in patients with suspected abscess a 6–8 hour postinjection scan is not totally reliable in excluding an inflammatory lesion. In the acutely ill patient or one who cannot undergo bowel preparation, we generally scan at 6–8 hours after injection and repeat the scan at 24 hours if possible. In patients who are less ill, and in whom it is believed that clinically a 24-hour wait will not be damaging, we omit the 6-hour image and prepare the bowel with a combination of laxatives for scanning at 24 hours. It is not uncommon in our laboratory to also obtain a scan at 48 hours when clear-cut clinical findings cannot be established on earlier studies.

Artifacts

Gallium-67 is taken up in areas of recent tissue disruption, for example, surgical wounds. We have found relatively little interference, however, from uptake in such sites, because they are generally recognizable and identifiable as such (Figure 1). Oblique views are helpful to demonstrate areas that are obscured by the incision site.

Instrumentation

We have found the scintillation camera to be far superior to the rectilinear scanner for use in patients with suspected inflammatory disease. Currently available multi-pulse height analyzer instruments with collimation tailored especially for gallium are particularly helpful (see Chapter 2). It is not uncommon for postoperative patients with suspected abscesses to have multiple surgical drains, tubes, and intravenous lines and be otherwise immobilized and uncomfortable. The flexibility of the scintillation camera allows imaging of multiple regions from various angles without moving the patient. The newer triple-window large-field cameras are not only more flexible but also require less imaging time than do the rectilinear scanners.

The majority of our patients are imaged on a moving table, large field of view, scintillation camera system. Suspicious areas are spot filmed at the conclusion of the total body scan. We have also found data processing particularly useful in images obtained during the first 24 hours postinjection. The lesion to background activity ratio is often low during this period. The lesion can be made more easily detectable by using the computer to subtract background in combination with a mild foreground enhancement.

The usual dose of gallium used for detection of inflammatory lesions is 3–5 mCi. However, higher doses, up to 10 mCi, have been recommended for tumor detection (see Chapter 7). Doses in the 8-mCi range may also be reasonable for abscess imaging, because the radiation dose is not excessive and because sensitivity, that is, appropriate count density, is important in lesion detectability (see Chapter 2).

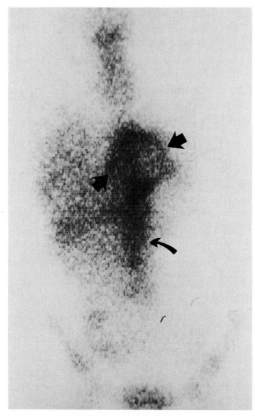

Figure 1.   Gallium scan (24 hour) in a febrile patient after resection of the left lobe of the liver for hemangioma. The circular area of increased uptake (large arrowhead) was identified overlying the operative site. The appearance of a rim of activity with a relatively "cold" center was much more suggestive of an inflammatory process, and this patient ultimately drained 300 cm^3 of pus from this site. The surgical incision (curved arrow) is readily identifiable and does not significantly interfere with interpretation of the scan.

INTRA-ABDOMINAL LESIONS: GENERAL CONSIDERATIONS

Since gallium imaging is sensitive for detection of inflammatory lesions and can usually identify the lesion within 24 hours of injection, it should be considered as a *primary* test in the diagnosis of abdominal sepsis. Nonetheless, it is always desirable to obtain a liver-spleen scan immediately prior to administration of gallium. A liver abscess is always a diagnostic possibility in any patient with abdominal sepsis, and gallium uptake in a liver abscess may be no greater than in the surrounding liver. Therefore, a "normal"-appearing liver on a gallium scan cannot be assumed to have excluded a hepatic abscess unless the colloid liver scan is also normal.

Conventional radiographic studies described in the previous chapter should also be obtained. While these studies are less sensitive than gallium scanning, they are quick and occasionally pathognomonic. Also, the radiographs may help determine if suspicious areas of gallium activity are within the displaced bowel. Oral or rectal administration of ^{99m}Tc-sulfur colloid can also be used for this purpose.

Ultrasonography should be attempted early. It is a rapid and effective method of detecting formed abscesses. Unfortunately, patients with abdominal abscesses frequently have marked distention with air-filled bowel that interferes with the ultrasonic examination. Often, a gallium-"directed" ultrasound examination will reveal a lesion that would be otherwise considered equivocal.

Computed tomography (CT) has not been in use long enough to determine its exact role in detecting abdominal abscesses. However, it is technically difficult to examine the entire abdomen by this technique. It is therefore preferable to withhold the CT study in patients without regional localizing signs or symptoms until some other study, such as the gallium scan, defines specific region to be evaluated. Radiographic, ultrasound, and CT methods can only detect a formed lesion. The gallium scan, however, may demonstrate an area of inflammation prior to frank abscess formation. Therefore, a positive gallium scan should not be disregarded, even if other "confirmatory" tests are normal.

Inflammatory Liver Disease

The patient with an intrahepatic abscess is at significant risk. The overall mortality in patients with hepatic abscesses is reported to be as high as 28%. In patients in whom the abscess is adequately treated, that is, by surgical drainage, followed by antibiotic therapy, the mortality drops to 4% (8). This disease is also associated with long hospitalizations. It is obvious that detection and adequate localization are absolutely essential and that the high initial cost of early diagnosis is far outweighed by both the human and economic costs of delayed or missed diagnosis.

The ^{99m}Tc-sulfur colloid liver scan should be the primary examination in patients with suspected hepatic abscess. However, a positive liver scan is not specific. Once a lesion is detected on a liver scan, a gallium scan may be very helpful in further refining the differential diagnosis. Gallium is not taken up in cysts, hemangiomas, and most pseudotumors of cirrhosis. Even with the gallium scan, however, it may not be possible to differentiate an acute hepatic inflammatory process from metastatic disease, multicentric hepatoma, or adenoma (9). The combination of the gallium scan and clinical picture may be sufficient to establish the diagnosis in some cases (Figure 2), while in others, radiographs, ultrasound, and CT studies may be required. As previously noted, the liver and gallium scans are helpful in defining the approximate region in which the ultrasound examination and/or the CT images should be obtained. Gallium-positive hepatic lesions that are complex (mixed) or sonolucent and have density readings below that of surrounding liver tissue are usually abscesses, whereas gallium-positive lesions that are solid and have density readings about equal to that of surrounding tissue are often tumors. Unfortunately, there are exceptions to these general patterns.

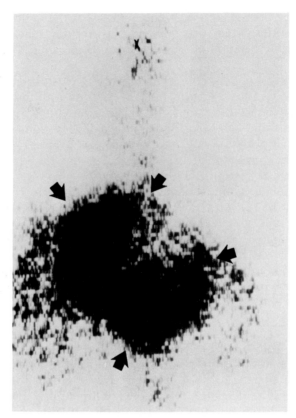

Figure 2.   Gallium scan (72 hour) in a patient admitted for complaints of epigastric fullness after an episode of pancreatitis. Note the large area of increased uptake (arrowheads) overlying the left lobe of the liver. At surgery, this area was found to be a pyogenic abscess of the liver.

Amebic Abscess

The gallium scan appearance of the acute hepatic amebic abscess has been characterized in the literature as a peripheral shell of increased uptake surrounding a cold central cavity (10). The rim of uptake has been correlated with an area of hyperemia noted histologically and arteriographically. Unfortunately, the sign is not specific for amebic abscess and may also be seen in large hepatic or retrohepatic abscesses and tumors as well (11) (Figure 3). The rim sign is somewhat analogous to the donut sign described in brain scanning. Gallium does not penetrate into the avascular portion of the abscess or into the necrotic central portion of the tumor.

Actinomycosis

A case has been reported of a patient with hepatic actinomycosis and focal abnormalities on a ^{99m}Tc-sulfur colloid liver scan. The gallium scan in this patient demonstrated increased concentration in the hepatic lesions (12). We have

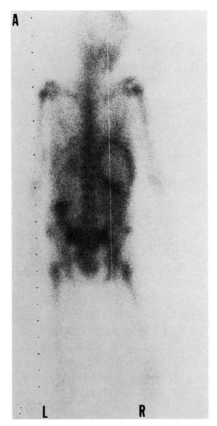

Figure 3A.   Moving table gallium scan (24 hour, posterior view) of a patient whose colon interposition distal anastomosis broke down. The patient was febrile, and, on gallium scan, a large "cold" area with a "hot" rim was seen in the region of the posterior liver.

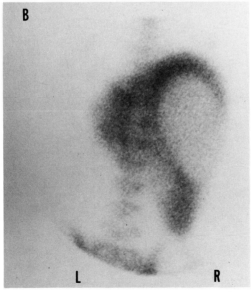

Figure 3B.   99mTc-sulfur colloid scan in the posterior projection shows an impression on the liver in the retrohepatic region. At surgery, a large retrohepatic abscess was found and drained.

seen a similar case of pulmonary actinomycosis in which gallium uptake was so intense that the normal features of liver uptake were not visible on the scan (Figure 4).

Cholangitis

Cholangitis may result in diffusely increased gallium uptake in one lobe of the liver. The ^{99m}Tc-sulfur colloid scan in such cases may be normal or show multiple areas of decreased uptake.

Gallbladder

Gallium has been employed for the diagnosis of empyema of the gallbladder. A study of four patients with empyema of the gallbladder reported by Lomas and Wagner in 1972 revealed that all had increased gallium uptake in the lesion (4). Unfortunately, the gallium scan is not useful in differentiating empyema from carcinoma of the gallbladder (Figures 5 & 6). While patients with acute cholecystitis, as expected, show increased gallium uptake in and around the gallbladder, only about 20% of patients with chronic cholecystitis exhibit any significant gal-

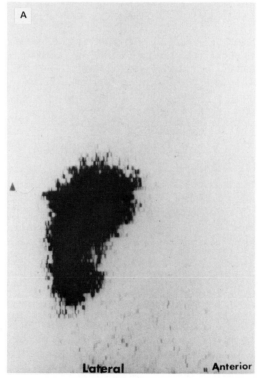

Figure 4A. Right lateral gallium scan demonstrates an intense area of increased uptake located posteriorly in the chest. Note that the liver directly beneath the area of uptake is barely visible due to the intense uptake in the lesion.

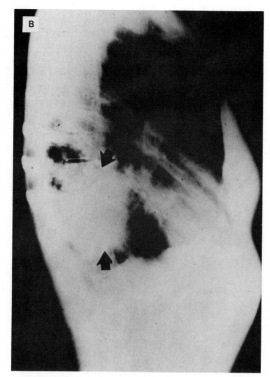

Figure 4B.   Chest x-ray lateral view in the same patient demonstrates an infiltrate posteriorly (arrowheads). At surgery, this lesion was resected and proved to be actinomycosis of the lung.

lium accumulation. Confusion of gallbladder uptake with the hepatic flexure is possible when bowel preparation is inadequate (13).

DETECTION OF SUBPHRENIC ABSCESSES WITH GALLIUM

The subphrenic abscess is one of the most feared complications of surgery (8,14). The anatomic features of this disease are discussed in Chapter 4. The nuclear medicine examination of choice in the diagnosis of the right subdia-phragmatic abscess is the combined liver-lung scan or liver-transmission scan (1). It should be stressed that when a combined liver-lung scan is performed, it should include a complete ^{99m}Tc-sulfur colloid liver scan prior to the injection of the lung-scanning agent. This precaution is taken to differentiate an intrahepa-tic abscess from a subphrenic lesion, because the clinical presentation of these two diseases may be identical. The specificity of liver-lung scanning is somewhat limited. It can be substantially improved by the addition of gallium scanning to the diagnostic evaluation (Figure 7).

Some investigators feel that a single set of images obtained 6–8 hours after injection is sufficient to determine the presence of a subphrenic abscess (7). Based on our previously mentioned experience in occasionally detecting absces-ses on later views only and the dire consequences of a missed diagnosis, we

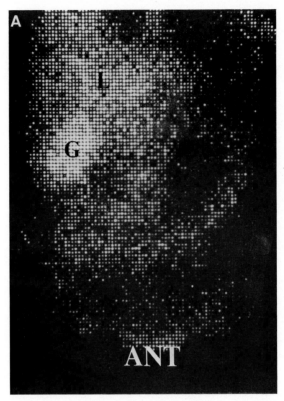

Figure 5A and 5B.   Computer-processed gallium scan of the liver 24 hours postinjection (anterior and RAO projections). There is intense increased uptake over the region of the gallbladder (G), as compared with the liver parentchyma (L). Repeat scans taken 48 hours after further bowel preparation showed no change in the configuration of this activity, thought to be within the gallbladder. At surgery, a carcinoma of the gallbladder was resected.

prefer to image at 6–8 hours and repeat the study, if it is negative or equivocal, at 24 hours.

Small subdiaphragmatic abscesses may be difficult to detect by the liver-lung scanning technique, because the separation between the two organs may be less than the resolution of the imaging system. Detection of small abscesses by the gallium scan is also difficult. The image of the liver may merge with the abscess and be overlooked. To avoid this problem, a dual-isotope subtraction method can be used to subtract the liver image from the gallium scan. This procedure results in increased visibility of gallium uptake in the right subdiaphragmatic space (15) (Figure 8). We feel that this method may be of benefit in patients suspected of harboring a right subdiaphragmatic abscess and in whom no lesion is detectable on the unprocessed gallium image.

Evaluation of the left subdiaphragmatic space by the gallium scan is potentially difficult, because activity in the spleen or splenic flexure of the colon may simulate a subdiaphragmatic lesion (7). Activity in this region is also noted in the immediate postsurgical period after splenectomy. It is especially marked in patients who have undergone splenectomy associated with laparotomy for lym-

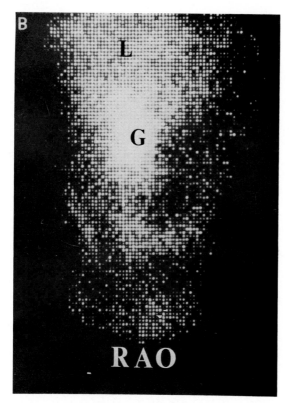

Figure 5, continued.

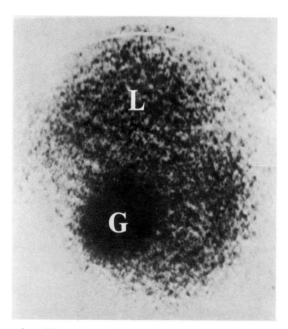

Figure 6. Right anterior oblique view of the hepatic region reveals marked increase in gallium uptake in the gallbladder (G), as compared with the liver parenchyma (L). This patient had acute cholecystitis. The scan findings are identical to those seen in the patient with carcinoma of the gallbladder described in Figures 5A and 5B.

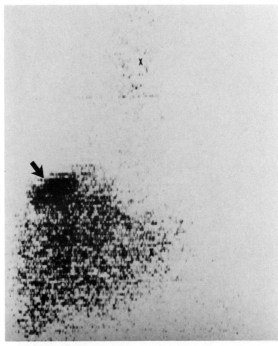

Figure 7.   This patient with chronic lymphocytic leukemia presented with fever and a peripheral blood smear that was more consistent with inflammatory disease than with recurrence of his leukemia. A 24-hour gallium scan demonstrated a localized area of increased uptake at the dome of the liver (arrow). Before surgery could be performed, this abscess ruptured through the diaphragm and drained through the lung.

phoma staging. The reason for this increased activity is not known. In spite of these problems, the gallium scan is still one of the few useful tools for detecting small inflammatory lesions in this area.

OTHER SITES OF INFLAMMATORY DISEASE OF THE ABDOMEN

There appears to be no significant difference between the accuracy of detection of visceral and nonvisceral abscesses within the abdomen by gallium scanning. Diffuse pancreatitis as well as infected pancreatic pseudocysts and free collections of pus have been identified on gallium scans (16–18) (Figures 9 & 10).

In a reported case of an infected pancreatic pseudocyst, the gallium scan was more specific than was diagnostic ultrasound. Ultrasonography demonstrated the cystic nature of the lesion but did not suggest the presence of infection. The gallium scan established the inflammatory nature of the lesion (17). This is only one small example of how combined use of various radiographic techniques improves specificity.

Although activity in the colon is often observed on gallium scans, it is not always a normal finding. Increased gallium uptake in the bowel wall occurs in pseudomembranous colitis (19). Scans performed within 24 hours after injection

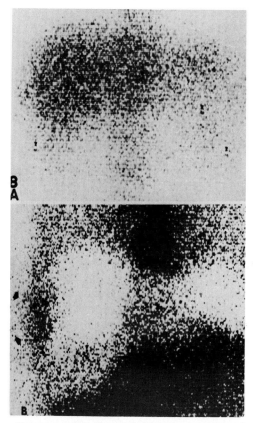

Figure 8.   A 24-hour gallium scan of the liver (A). Dual-isotope subtraction technique (B) demonstrates a localized area of increased gallium uptake (arrowheads) at the right border of the liver. This area corresponded to a localized inflammatory site.

usually show relatively little bowel activity. The appearance of persistent bowel activity with no change after enemas or laxatives should alert the observer to the possible presence of inflammatory bowel disease. Persistent localized bowel activity may occur in regional enteritis and diverticulitis of the colon (20) (Figure 11).

The overall sensitivity and specifity of gallium-67 imaging in detecting abdominal abscesses is described in Table 1 on page 90.

Postoperative Uptake of Gallium in the Region of the Pancreas

In postoperative patients, especially those who have undergone surgery in or around the pancreas, it has been our experience that there is a diffuse inflammatory reaction that results and simulates the appearance of an abscess (Figure 12). This reaction may be due to leakage of pancreatic enzymes and the resultant inflammatory reaction that these enzymes produce. The uptake may persist, even after the patient is totally asymptomatic. On surgical reexploration of these patients, little, if any, pus is identified. The reaction is probably similar to that of a cellulitis with no localized pus collection.

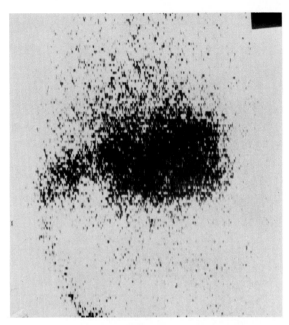

Figure 9.   A 6-hour gallium scan of the liver region demonstrates a diffuse area of increased uptake in the midabdomen not thought to be within the liver. The patient was recently explored for common bile duct stones. At postmortem examination, a large free intra-abdominal abscess was found at the site of increased uptake.

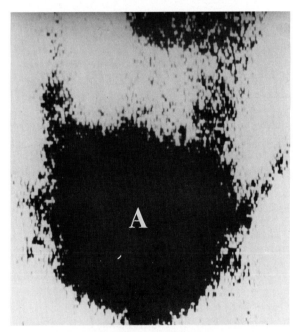

Figure 10.   A 32-year-old white male after resection of distal colon for carcinoma became markedly febrile. Gallium scan of the abdomen demonstrated a massive area of increased uptake (A) in the pelvis, which at surgery proved to be a large pelvic abscess.

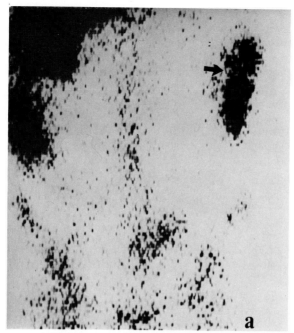

Figure 11A. Patient with a fever of unknown origin who was studied for an occult abscess. An area of increased uptake (arrow) was noted overlying the descending colon. There was no change in the appearance of this area on 48-hour scans, and the differential diagnosis included inflammatory bowel disease and diverticulitis.

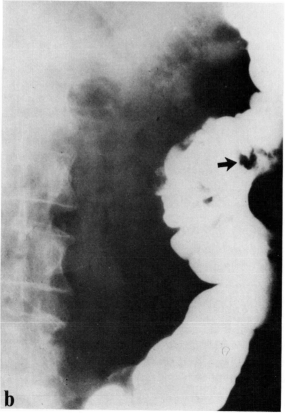

Figure 11B. Barium enemas in the same patient demonstrate irregularity in the corresponding region of the descending colon (arrow) due to fissuring in a region of diverticulitis.

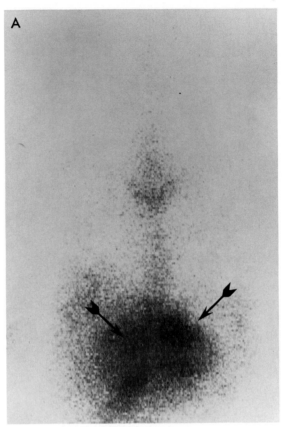

Figure 12A.   This patient developed fever after a Whipple procedure. The 24-hour gallium scan revealed a large area of increased uptake (arrow) overlying the surgical site and extending considerably beyond it. Diagnosis of intra-abdominal abscess was made, and the patient was reexplored. Only 50 cm³ of pus and a diffuse inflammatory reaction were discovered.

Pelvis   Especially careful bowel preparation is required to evaluate suspected pelvic lesions, because retained activity in the rectum is commonly seen. Also, bladder activity is frequently observed on 6- and 24-hour images. Therefore, it is necessary that the patient void as completely as possible prior to imaging the pelvic region.

Retroperitoneum   Gallium scanning is the only nuclear medicine procedure that plays an important primary role in the diagnosis of retroperitoneal abscesses. The recommended protocol for suspected inflammatory disease in the retroperitoneal and intraperitoneal regions is similar to that for the hepatic and perihepatic regions. Severely ill patients should be studied 6–8 hours after gallium injection. If the initial scan is negative, rescanning at 24 hours after injection may increase the detection yield. Since early gallium scanning results in a high background of gallium, and consequently in a low target to nontarget ratio, we recommend a scintillation camera and a data-processing device for background subtraction, if available.

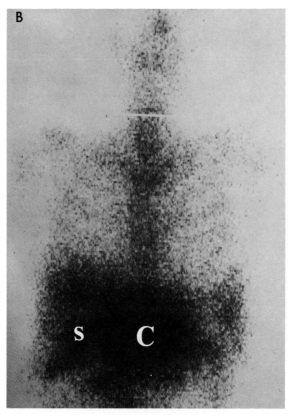

Figure 12B. Same patient 6 weeks after operation with remaining intense increased uptake over the previous area of inflammation (C) and linearly increased uptake over a drain site (S). At this point, the patient was completely afebrile.

Renal Disease

The signs and symptoms of renal inflammatory disease may at times be confused with those of an intra-abdominal abscess. Although radiographic techniques, such as fluoroscopy and intravenous excretory urography, are well established, they may still fail to detect a perinephric abscess. In a series of patients studied 6 hours after injection of gallium, all perinephric abscesses were correctly localized. In two of the cases, the intravenous pyelograms, nephrotomograms, ultrasound, and renal angiography were normal (21). It is useful to identify the exact location of the kidney when a perinephric lesion is suspected. ^{99m}Technetium-iron ascorbate or ^{99m}Tc-DMSA may be used for this purpose and can also be utilized for subtraction studies analogous to the liver subtraction method previously described.

It is not uncommon to see bilateral symmetric renal uptake on the 24-hour gallium scan. In a review of 175 gallium scans in patients without malignancy, renal activity was noted in 7% of this group at 48 hours (22). The nonneoplastic

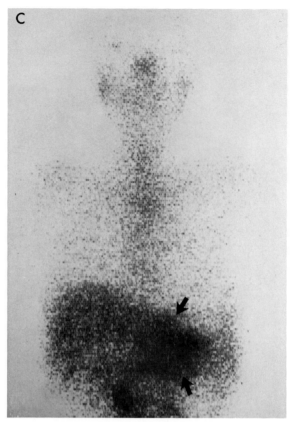

Figure 12C.   Four months after operation, there remains a significant area of increased uptake overlying the previous inflammatory site (arrows). At this time, the patient is totally asymptomatic.

causes for renal uptake include pyelonephritis, acute tubular necrosis, renal vasculitis, interstitial nephritis, and renal abscess.

The appearance of intense uptake in the kidney is certainly worthy of persistent investigation to the point of renal biopsy. More than 80% of patients with pyelonephritis will have positive gallium scans (23) (Figure 13). Frequently, patients with pyelonephritis who present clinically with fever and abdominal pain are suspected of having an intra-abdominal inflammatory lesion. The appearance of a "hot" kidney on a gallium scan can establish the correct diagnosis. This is one situation in which the use of gallium may save the patient from an exploratory laparotomy for an occult abscess.

In patients with known malignancies, the uptake within the kidney has a somewhat different connotation. In the series reported from the National Institutes of Health, the vast majority of patients with renal uptake on gallium scan later than 24 hours and with known primary malignancies had an infiltrative tumor in the kidneys (24). Bekerman and Vias have reported two cases of patients with renal amyloidosis who also had prominent gallium uptake in the kidneys (25).

To reiterate, bilateral renal uptake that persists significantly after 24 hours requires further intensive evaluation (Figure 14).

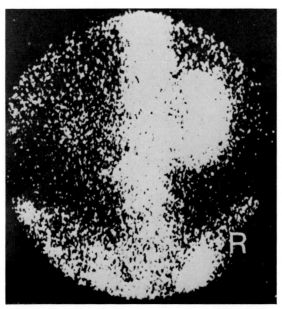

Figure 13.   Scintillation camera posterior view of the renal region on a gallium scan. There is increased uptake in the right kidney. The diagnosis of pyelonephritis was subsequently established.

Renal Transplants

The group of patients undergoing renal transplantation presents a special set of problems with relation to gallium scanning. The altered immune state of these patients makes them somewhat more susceptible to infectious processes. Paradoxically, gallium scanning is slightly less efficient in detecting inflammatory disease in these patients, probably due also to their immunosuppressed status.

When evaluating patients after renal transplantation, one may occasionally identify the transplanted kidney. Significant gallium accumulation in the kidney may occur with either rejection or acute tubular necrosis (26,27). The normally functioning kidney transplant does not accumulate gallium. [The behavior of gallium appears to be similar to that of ^{99m}Tc-sulfur colloid and radiolabeled fibrinogen. All of these agents may accumulate in rejecting kidneys (26).] Therefore, in evaluating the renal transplant patient for an infectious process, the appearance of gallium within the kidney must be correlated with the functional state of that kidney.

NONABDOMINAL INFLAMMATORY DISEASE

Chest

The principle diagnostic tool for evaluating pulmonary inflammatory disease is, and will continue to be, the chest radiograph. However, there are certain specific situations in which the gallium scan may be of value in either establishing a diagnosis or evaluating the effects of treatment.

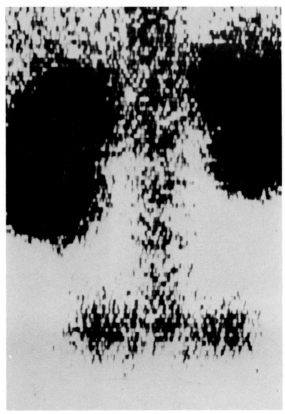

Figure 14.   A 48-hour postinjection gallium scan. Intense increased uptake is noted in both kidneys. The patient was 6 weeks postoperation for a cervical conization, when her blood urea nitrogen level began to rise significantly. The bilateral uptake seen within both kidneys suggested a diffuse infammatory process of the kidneys. Renal biopsy established the diagnosis of drug-induced interstitial nephritis.

Pneumocystis carinii

Pneumocystis carinii is an opportunistic organism responsible for producing interstitial pneumonitis in infants. It also may produce pneumonia in older children and adults who are being treated with cytotoxic and/or immunosuppressive medications. Its onset is insidious, and its consequences are often devastating. Levenson and associates (28) described two patients with *P. carinii* in whom marked lung uptake of gallium was observed in the absence of marked radiographic changes. They indicate that pulmonary uptake of ^{67}Ga that is disproportionate to chest radiographic changes in a patient receiving chemotherapy or immunosuppressant drugs is suggestive of *P. carinii* infection, and they recommend lung biopsy to confirm the diagnosis if clinically indicated.

Pneumoconiosis

The pattern of gallium uptake in pneumoconiosis is rather diffuse and nonspecific. However, it is suggested that gallium scanning might be useful in detecting the early stages of this disease. It has been shown that when overt radiographic changes are present, there is significant gallium uptake. There is some reason to believe that it may be useful to study the activity and progression of the disease with gallium (29).

Sarcoidosis

A study by Heshiki and colleagues revealed that 61% of patients with mild to severe parenchymal infiltrates due to sarcoidosis concentrated gallium (30). In no case did gallium accumulate in radiographically normal regions of the lung. In patients who were studied during a relapse of the disease, two thirds displayed increased gallium uptake. However, approximately 25% of the patients with clinically progressive disease showed no gallium uptake.

When the accumulation of gallium in hilar nodes was studied, virtually all patients had gallium-positive nodes. Nearly half of those with positive gallium scans, however, had no evidence of adenopathy on chest x-ray. A small subgroup of these patients was treated with steroids for between 5 and 7 months. There was no improvement in the appearance of the chest x-ray. However, the gallium scans did show improvement with resolution of areas of abnormal uptake. The scan findings correlated well with the patients' clinical status. The authors concluded that gallium scanning may be of some value in following patients undergoing steroid therapy for sarcoidosis (30,31) (Figure 15). The detection of systemic sarcoid by gallium scanning is also possible. Its appearance at times may simulate a lymphoma (Figure 16).

Idiopathic Pulmonary Fibrosis

Idiopathic pulmonary fibrosis is an evolutionary disease process that begins with lung injury from any of a number of causes and progresses from an alveolitis stage to fibrosis with subsequent honey-combing. X-rays and perfusion and ventilation scans may be useful in documenting the pulmonary damage in regions of the lung that have reached the end stages of the disease process, but they are not useful for monitoring the active inflammatory stages. Line and associates (32,33) have shown that gallium uptake in the lung correlates well with the activity of the disease, as reflected in the number of neutrophils present in pulmonary lavage fluid. They advocate the use of a "gallium index" to document the activity of the disease. The gallium index takes into account both the intensity and the pattern of gallium uptake in the lung.

Gallium will concentrate in other inflammatory lung diseases, including tuberculosis and pyogenic pneumonias, and has been suggested as a method to differentiate pulmonary infarct from pneumonia (34,35). Bleomycin pulmonary toxicity also results in diffuse bilateral pulmonary uptake of [67]Ga. The pulmonary uptake decreases after treatment (36).

Central Nervous System

While gallium does accumulate in inflammatory lesions within and adjacent to the brain, it is not generally useful for detection or differentiation of such lesions. Waxman and Siemsen compared the sensitivity of gallium citrate and

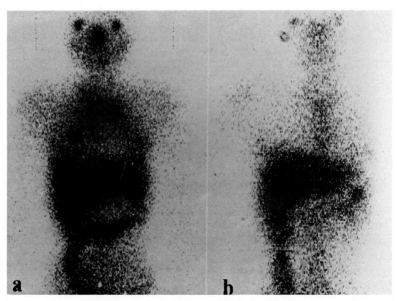

Figure 15.   Pretreatment film in a patient with sarcoidosis (A). Note the intense increased uptake over the hilar region and parenchymal uptake. After treatment with steroids (B), there is virtually complete clearing of the parenchymal and nodal uptake.

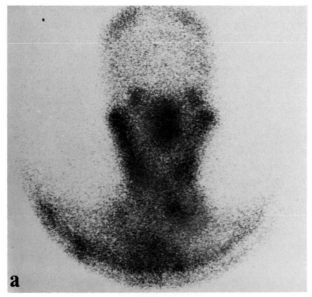

Figure 16A.   A 23-year-old female with known systemic sarcoidosis. Scintillation camera spot view of the head and neck shows markedly increased uptake in the cervical lymph nodes, nasopharynx, and left supraclavicular region. Parotid gland uptake is also identified.

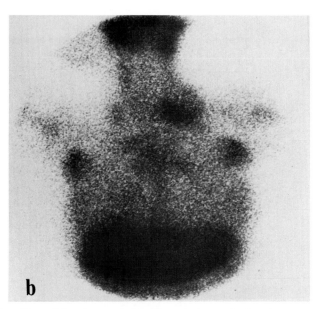

Figure 16B.   Spot films of the chest region in the anterior projection demonstrate left and right supraclavicular, mediastinal, and axillary uptake. There is relatively little uptake over the chest, corresponding to the normal radiographic findings in this patient's chest. Other spot views indicated periaortic, inguinal, and iliac node involvement.

99mTc pertechnetate imaging for the diagnosis of infections in and around the brain. The gallium scan detected all five intracerebral abscesses in their series, whereas the conventional brain scan detected only three of the five lesions (37). However, their study involved only a small group of patients and did not compare results with computed tomography. In our experience, the combination of conventional radionuclide brain imaging with either 99mTc pertechnetate or 99mTc-DTPA and computed tomography has an overall sensitivity of 96% for all intracranial lesions, including inflammatory disease. The gallium scan would be useful, therefore, in only rare instances where an inflammatory lesion was strongly suspected clinically but not detected by other means.

The gallium scan is also probably not useful in categorizing intracranial lesions. It is positive not only in inflammatory disease and tumor but probably also in cerebral infarction (38,39), although this point is still somewhat controversial (40).

Bone and Joint

The early diagnosis of osteomyelitis is an important clinical problem. The disease occurs primarily in children and young adults. It is especially common in drug abusers who use intravenous medications. Early diagnosis and treatment are important, because chronic lesions may produce deformity and become extremely refractory to antibiotic therapy.

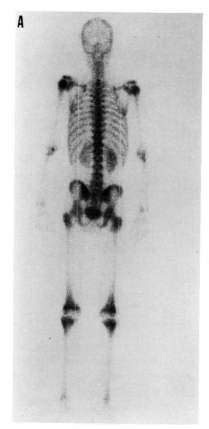

Figure 17A.   Normal bone scan in a 17-year-old patient with regional enteritis and intense low back pain.

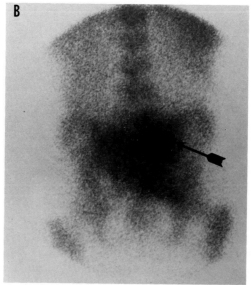

Figure 17B.   Posterior gallium scan of the pelvic region at 72 hours demonstrates a localized area of increased uptake that represents an early osteomyelitis secondary to a fistula from regional enteritis.

Handmaker and Giammona have discussed the use of gallium in septic arthritis (41). They have found that the gallium scan will usually be positive in the septic arthridities at a time when the bone scan is still negative. Early uptake of gallium in osteomyelitis with a negative bone scan also occurs early in the disease process. Therefore, the findings of a normal x-ray, normal bone scan, and abnormal gallium scan in the region of a bone or joint are entirely consistent with septic arthritis, and prompt treatment is indicated.

The pattern of a positive gallium scan with a normal bone scan is not restricted to primary bone and joint infections but may also occur when inflammatory lesions invade bone from an adjacent location (Figure 17).

The normal appearance of the bone scan in some cases of early osteomyelitis is probably due to a compromise of local vascularity. This phenomenon may occur as a result of a septic embolus in a major intraosseous vessel or as a result of elevated pressure within the bone due to bacterial growth and pus formation. The gallium scan is not only useful in establishing the diagnosis of osteomyelitis but probably also in monitoring treatment.

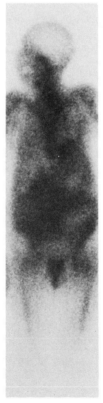

Figure 18.   Gallium uptake in an area of recent myocardial infarction. Gallium was administered for detection of a suspected postoperative abscess. The patient developed severe chest pain a few hours after injection. The infarct was confirmed by pyrophosphate, electrocardiogram, and enzyme changes. The scan was performed 72 hours after injection. The diminished liver activity is related to polycystic disease of that organ.

TABLE 1   [67]Ga UPTAKE IN ABDOMINAL ABSCESS

	Positive Scan / Proven Abscess	Negative Scan / No Abscess	Other Inflammatory Lesions Detected
Kumar (43) 1977	13/15	19/20	15/15
Shimshak (44) 1977	8/8	5/7	
Caffee (45) 1977	12/14	30/37	
Hopkins (46) 1976	52/56	61/64	20/20
Damron (47) 1976	15/15	36/36	
Kumar (20) 1975	21/21	11/11	4/4
Habibian (48) 1975	4/4	5/5	6/6
Harvey (49) 1975	22/29	37/39	
Teates (50) 1975	10/13	22/26	3/3
Fratkin (51) 1974	15/17	7/7	
Littenberg (5) 1973	5/5	1/1	6/6
TOTAL	177/197 (90%)	234/253 (92%)	54/54

Myocardial Infarction

Since there is muscle infiltration with leukocytes immediately after myocardial infarction, the role of gallium in detecting this disease entity has been evaluated. Unfortunately, the lesion to background ratio of gallium activity is low, typically about 2:1. By comparison, technetium diphosphonate and polyphosphate compounds have 16:1 and 28:1 lesion to background ratios, respectively. The level of gallium uptake in infarcts is usually insufficient for imaging of these lesions on a routine clinical basis (42) (Figure 18).

CONCLUSIONS

We have presented a rather detailed discussion of the use of gallium in the detection of inflammatory disease. Although ^{67}Ga citrate has been used for evaluation of inflammatory disease for only a few years, more than 50% of the gallium studies currently performed in our laboratory are for detection of occult inflammatory processes. We anticipate this proportion to remain about the same or increase slightly in the future.

The cooperative efforts of many disciplines have increased the specificity of the findings on gallium scans. Careful attention to details of scanning and bowel preparation will yield a high number of true-positive studies. A knowledge of the pitfalls involved in gallium scanning in terms of nonsurgical causes of positive scans, such as regional enteritis and pyelonephritis, will result in improved patient care and growing physician confidence in the use of gallium scanning.

REFERENCES

1.   Briggs RC: Combined liver-lung scanning in detecting subdiaphragmatic abscess. *Sem Nucl Med* **2**:150, 1972.

2.   Edwards CL, Hayes RL: Tumor scanning with 67 gallium citrate. *J Nucl Med* **10**:103, 1969.

3.   Lavender JP, Loew J, Barker JR, et al: Gallium-67 citrate scanning in neoplastic and inflammatory lesions. *Brit J Radiol* **11**:361, 1971.

4.   Lomas F, Wagner HN Jr: Accumulation of ionic 67 gallium in empyema of the gallbladder. *Radiology* **105**:689, 1972.

5. Littenberg RL, Taketa RM, Alazraki NP, et al: Gallium-67 for localization of septic lesions. *Ann Intern Med* **79**:403, 1973.

6. Sanders RC, James AE Jr, Fischer K: Correlation of liver scans and images with abdominal radiographs in perihepatic sepsis. *Amer J Surg* **124**:346, 1972.

7. Hopkins GB, Mende CW: Gallium-67 and subphrenic abscesses, is delayed scintigraphy necessary? *J Nucl Med* **16**:609, 1975.

8. Altemeier WA, Culbertson WR, Fullen WD, et al: Intra-abdominal abscesses. *Amer J Surg* **125**:70, 1973.

9. Belanger MA, Beauchamp JM, Neitzschman HR: Gallium uptake in benign tumor of the liver: case report. *J Nucl Med* **15**:470, 1975.

10. Geslien GE, Thrall JH, Johnson MC: Gallium scanning in acute hepatic amoebic abscess. *J Nucl Med* **15**:561, 1975.

11. DeRoo MJK: Scintigraphic appearance of necrotic liver metastasis identical with that of amoebic abscesses. *J Nucl Med* **16**:250, 1975.

12. Chandarlapaty SKC, Dusol M, Edwards R, et al: Gallium-67 accumulation in hepatic actinomycosis. *Gastroenterology* **59**:752, 1975.

13. Waxman AD, Siemsen JK: Gallium gallbladder scanning in cholecystitis. *J Nucl Med* **16**:148, 1975.

14. Sherman NJ, David JR, Jesseph HE: Subphrenic abscess, a continuing hazard. *Amer J Surg* **117**:117, 1969.

15. Damron JR, Beihn RM, Selby JB, et al: Gallium-technetium subtraction scanning for the localization of subphrenic abscess. *Radiology* **113**:117, 1974.

16. Hopkins GB, Kan M, Mende CW: Early 67 gallium scintigraphy for the localization of abdominal abscesses. *J Nucl Med* **16**:990, 1975.

17. Kennedy TD, Martin NL, Robinson RG, et al: Identification of an infected pseudocyst of the pancreas with 67 gallium citrate: case report. *J Nucl Med* **16**:1132, 1975.

18. Fratkin MJ, Sharpe AR Jr: Non-tuberculous psoas abscess: localization using 67-gallium. *J Nucl Med* **14**:499, 1973.

19. Tedesco FJ, Coleman E, Siegel BA: Gallium 67 accumulation in pseudomembranous colitis. *J Amer Med Ass* **235**:1, 1976.

20. Kumar B, Coleman RE, Alderson PO: Gallium 67 citrate imaging in patients with suspected inflammatory processes. *Arch Surg* **110**:1237, 1975.

21. Kessler WO, Gittes RF, Hurwitz SR, et al: Gallium-67 scans in the diagnosis of pyelonephritis. *West J Med* **121**:91, 1973.

22. Kumar B, Coleman RE: Significance of delayed 67 gallium localization in the kidneys. *J Nucl Med* **17**:872, 1976.

23. Hurwitz SR, Kessler WO, Alazraki NP, et al: Gallium-67 imaging to localize urinary tract infections. *Brit J Radiol* **49**:156, 1976.

24. Frankel RS, Richman SD, Levenson SM, et al: Renal localization of gallium 67 citrate. *Radiology* **114**:393, 1975.

25. Bekerman C, Vias M: Renal localization of 67 gallium citrate in renal amyloidosis: case report. *J Nucl Med* **17**:899, 1976.

26. George EA, Codd JE, Newton WT, et al: Comparative evaluation of renal transplant rejection with radioiodinated fibrinogen, 99m-Tc S.C. or gallium citrate. *J Nucl Med* **17**:175, 1976.

27. George EA, Codd JE, Newton WT, et al: 67-Gallium citrate in renal allograft of rejection. *Radiology* **117**:731, 1975.

28. Levenson SM, Warren RD, Richman SD, et al: Abnormal pulmonary gallium accumulation in P. carinii pneumonia. *Radiology* **119**:395, 1976.

29. Siemsen JR, Sargent EN, Grebe SF, et al: Pulmonary concentration of gallium 67 in pneumoconiosis. *Amer J Roentgenol Radium Ther Nucl Med* **120**:815, 1974.

30. Heshiki A, Schatz SL, McKusick KA, et al: Gallium-67 citrate scanning in patients with pulmonary sarcoidosis. *Amer J Roentgenol Radium Ther Nucl Med* **122**:744, 1974.

31. McKusick KA, Soin JS, Ghildai A, et al: Gallium 67 accumulation in pulmonary sarcoidosis. *J Amer Med Ass* **233**:688, 1973.

32. Crystal RG, Fulmer JD, Roberts WC, et al: Idiopathic pulmonary fibrosis, clinical, histologic, radiographic physiologic, scintigraphic and biochemical aspects. *Ann Intern Med* **85**:769, 1976.

33. Line BR, Fulmer JD, Jones AE, et al: [67]Gallium scanning in idiopathic pulmonary fibrosis: correlation with histopathology and bronchoalveolar lavage [Abstract]. *Amer Rev Resp Diseases* **113**:244, 1976.

34. Mishkin FS, Niden AH, Pick RA, et al: Gallium lung imaging as an aid in the differential diagnosis between pulmonary infarction and pneumonitis. *J Nucl Med* **16**:551, 1971.

35. Niden AH, Mishkin FS, Khurana MML, et al: [67]Ga lung scan, an aid in the differential diagnosis of pulmonary embolism and pneumonitis. *J Amer Med Ass* **237**:1206, 1977.

36. Richman SD, et al: [67]Ga accumulation in pulmonary lesions associated with bleomycin toxicity. *Cancer* **36**:1966, 1975.

37. Waxman AD, Siemsen JK: Gallium scanning of cranial and intracranial infections. *J Nucl Med* **16**:580, 1975.

38. Poulose RC, Reba RC, Goodyear M: Gallium-67 citrate and cerebral infarction. *Invest Radiol* **11**:20, 1976.

39. Wallner RJ, Croll MN, Brady LW: Gallium-67 localization in acute cerebral infarction. *J Nucl Med* **15**:308, 1974.

40. Waxman AD, Siemsen JK, Lee CL, et al: Reliability of gallium scanning in the detection and differentiation of central nervous system lesions. *Radiology* **116**:675, 1975.

41. Handmaker H, Giammona ST: "Hot joint"—increased diagnostic accuracy using combined 99m-Tc phosphate and 67 gallium citrate imaging in pediatrics *(abstract)*. *J Nucl Med* **17**:554, 1976.

42. Zweiman FG, Holeman BL, O'Keefe A, et al: Selective uptake of 99m-Tc complexes and 67 gallium in acutely infarcted myocardium. *J Nucl Med* **16**:975, 1975.

43. Kumar B, Alderson PO, Geisse G: The role of ^{67}Ga citrate imaging and diagnostic ultrasound in patients with suspected abdominal abscesses. *J Nucl Med* **18**:534, 1977.

44. Shimshak R, Korobkin M, Hoffer P, Hill T, Schor R, Kressel H: The complementary role of 67-Ga and CT scans for detection of abdominal inflammation. *J Nuc Med* **18**:636, 1977.

45. Caffee H, Watts G, Mena I: Gallium-citrate scanning in the diagnosis of intra-abdominal abscess. *Amer J Surg* **133**:665, 1977.

46. Hopkins GB, Kan M, Mende CN: Gallium-67 scintigraphy and infra-abdominal sepsis. *West J Med* **125**:425, 1976.

47. Damron JR, Beihn RM, Deland F: Detection of upper abdominal abscesses by radionuclide imaging. *Radiology* **120**:131, 1976.

48. Habibian MR, Staab EV, Matthews HA: Gallium citrate ^{67}Ga scans in febrile patients. *JAMA* **233**:1073, 1975.

49. Harvey WC, Podoloff DA, Kopp DT: Gallium-67 in 68 consecutive infection searches. *J Nucl Med* **16**:2, 1975.

50. Teates CD, Hunter JG, Jr.: Gallium scanning as a screening test for inflammatory lesions. *Radiology* **116**:383, 1975.

51. Fratkin MF, Hirsch JI, Sharpe AR, et al: Ga-67 localization of post-operative abdominal abscesses. *J Nucl Med* **15**:491, 1974.

Part 3

Neoplastic Diseases

7

Malignant Lymphoma

David A. Turner, M.D.

Associate Professor of Nuclear Medicine
and Radiology
Rush Medical College
Department of Nuclear Medicine
Rush-Presbyterian—St. Luke's Medical Center
Chicago, Illinois

Ernest W. Fordham, M.D.

Professor of Nuclear Medicine and Radiology
Rush Medical College
Chairman, Department of Nuclear Medicine
Rush-Presbyterian—St. Luke's Medical Center
Chicago, Illinois

Robert E. Slayton, M.D.

Associate Professor of Medicine
Rush Medical College
Department of Nuclear Medicine
Rush-Presbyterian—St. Luke's Medical Center
Chicago, Illinois

Opinion varies greatly regarding the usefulness of gallium-67 (^{67}Ga) scanning in the management of malignant lymphoma. Some investigators extol its virtues (1–8), while others, in informal conversation, reveal considerable disenchantment. These differences arise from anecdotal experiences, variation in imaging techniques, and differences in the clinical settings in which ^{67}Ga scanning is employed.

Gallium-67 is not an ideal tumor-scanning agent but, rather, an "all-purpose disease finder" that also localizes in inflamed tissues and certain normal organs. Hence, biopsy may be necessary to confirm the presence of tumor when a scan is positive.

When used to identify sites of lymphoma, the sensitivity of ^{67}Ga scanning is less than one might hope (applying criteria for scan interpretation that minimize the false-positive rate). However, if one takes reasonable steps to maximize image quality, ^{67}Ga scanning will be useful to the clinician in varying degrees, depending on the clinical problem in question.

CORRELATION OF DETECTABILITY WITH HISTOLOGIC TYPE OF LYMPHOMA

The sensitivity* of ^{67}Ga scanning in the detection of disease varies with the type of lymphoma (Table 1) (3,6–8), appearing to be greatest in Hodgkin's disease and the histiocytic lymphomas. Based on published reports, and using conservative criteria for interpretation of images, one may expect to detect about 70% of lesions in patients with these lymphomas. The sensitivity for lymphocytic and mixed lymphocytic-histiocytic lymphoma ranges from about 30 to 50%, with a false-positive rate† (FPR) of 5%.

CORRELATION OF DETECTABILITY WITH ANATOMIC SITE

Detectability of lymphomas with ^{67}Ga scanning varies with anatomic site (Table 2) (1–3,6–8). For example, masses that occur within or near the liver may be difficult to detect, because they are obscured by normal accumulation of activity by that organ (3). Some authors have suggested that superficial masses are easier to detect than those that are situated deep within the abdomen (3,6). Most observers find it relatively difficult to interpret the iliac nodal regions because of radioactivity in the overlying cecum and sigmoid colon, which may persist despite vigorous purging.

Detectability at a given site may also depend on histologic type. Turner et al. (3) and Johnston et al. (6) report that Hodgkin's disease is more easily detected in superficial sites than in abdominal sites. Greenlaw et al. (7) could find no differ-

$$*\text{Sensitivity} = \frac{\text{number of truly diseased sites positive on scan}}{\text{total number of truly diseased sites}} \times 100;$$

a constant false-positive rate is assumed.

$$†\text{False-positive rate} = \frac{\text{number of normal sites called positive}}{\text{total number of normal sites evaluated}} \times 100.$$

TABLE 1   RESULTS OF ^{67}Ga SCANNING VERSUS TYPE OF MALIGNANT
LYMPHOMA*

Type of Lymphoma	Series	Sensitivity (%)	False-positive Rate (%)
Hodgkin's disease	Turner et al. (3)	77	5
	Johnston et al. (6)	65	< 5[†]
Histiocytic lymphoma	Greenlaw et al. (7)	71	< 5[†]
	Levi et al. (8)	78	~ 5
Mixed-cell lymphoma	Greenlaw et al. (7)	53	< 5[†]
	Levi et al. (8)	46	~ 5
Lymphocytic (well and poorly differentiated)	Greenlaw et al. (7)	32	< 5[†]
	Levi et al. (8)	55	~ 5

*Except for the series of Levi et al., these data are based primarily on histologic confirma-
tion of the presence or absence of disease.
[†]The false-positive rate (FPR) as defined in the text could not be determined directly
from the data given by these authors. The FPR given here is an estimate based on Bayes'
theorem (see Appendix B).

ence when comparing sensitivities at these sites in the non-Hodgkin's lymphomas.

Apparent regional differences in the detectability of lesions may be related, in
part, to differences in the methods used to confirm the presence of disease. For
example, the presence or absence of abdominal lymphoma is generally
confirmed by biopsy at laparotomy, whereas the presence or absence of disease
in the mediastinum is usually "proved" by radiography, itself a relatively insensi-
tive technique. Even in series in which mediastinal disease has been proven
histologically, it is usually only radiographically apparent tumor masses that have
been biopsied. Hence, it is likely that patients who have large mediastinal lesions
will be correctly identified, whereas those with small lesions are thought to be
free of mediastinal disease. Since large lesions are more easily detected by scanning than are small ones (8), the sensitivity of ^{67}Ga scanning in detecting mediastinal disease appears to be higher than it is in actuality. It is clear, however, that
[67]Ga scanning is at least as sensitive as radiography for detecting mediastinal
lymphoma (1–3,6,8,9).

EFFECT OF IMPROVED IMAGING TECHNIQUES ON LESION DETECTABILITY

In all of the studies of the accuracy of ^{67}Ga scanning patients with malignant
lymphoma referred to above, patients were imaged with 5-in. dual probe rectilinear scanners (with variable pulse height analysis) after administration of
approximately 0.043 mCi/kg of ^{67}Ga citrate. Under these conditions, image
quality is severely limited by low maximum count densities [as low as 15–75

TABLE 2   RESULTS OF ^{67}Ga SCANS BY ANATOMIC REGIONS IN UNTREATED HODGKIN'S DISEASE AND NON-HODGKIN'S LYMPHOMA (histologically proven sites, except as indicated)

Series	Anatomic Site	True Positive	False Negative	True-positive Rate (%)	True Negative	False Positive	False-positive Rate (%)
Turner et al. (3) (Hodgkin's disease)	Mediastinum*	21	0	100	15	2	12
	Superficial lymph nodes	15	4	79	13	1	7
	Para-aortic mesenteric region	5	5	50	24	4	14
	Portal nodes	0	7	0	31	0	0
	Iliac nodes	0	5	0	69	2	3
	Spleen	7	2	78	24	5	17
	Liver	0	0	—	38	0	0
Johnston et al. (6) (Hodgkin's disease)	Neck	75	15	83	—	—	Overall false-positive rate of about 5% (see Appendix B)
	Thorax	15	1	94	—	—	
	Axilla	5	5	50	—	—	
	Abdominal-pelvic	57	58	50	—	—	
	Inguinofemoral	6	6	50	—	—	
Greenlaw et al. (7) (non-Hodgkin's lymphoma)	Neck	34	30	53	—	—	Overall false-positive rate of about 5% (see Appendix B)
	Thorax	7	2	78	—	—	
	Axilla	6	12	33	—	—	
	Abdominal-pelvic	60	66	48	—	—	
	Inguinofemoral	15	12	56	—	—	
Levi et al. (8) (non-Hodgkin's lymphoma)	Neck and axilla	15	6	71	1	0	0
	Thorax*	14	1	93	24	5	17
	Para-aortic mesenteric	22	1	96	18	0	0
	Pelvic-inguinal	9	9	50	30	0	0
	Liver	3	3	50	22	2	8
	Spleen	3	2	60	11	1	8

*Radiographic *or* histologic findings taken as proof of disease at site or lack thereof.

98

counts/cm² for scanning speeds of 700 cm/min (1)]. Furthermore, the spatial resolution of the medium-energy collimators usually used with rectilinear scanners for ^{67}Ga scanning falls off rapidly with distance from their geometric focal planes, so that the spatial resolution in the midcoronal plane of an average-sized adult will be very poor (of the order of 4 cm, full width at half maximum). Substantial improvement in image quality can be achieved if the count density is maximized by counting three peaks rather than one (see chapter 2) and by increasing the dose of ^{67}Ga used (2) (Figure 1). We administer 0.14 mCi/kg, up to a total dose of 10 mCi/kg, to patients with histologically proved lymphoma. The higher radiation dose (approximately 3.4 rads, whole body) is easily justified in these patients, who will receive radiation therapy and/or chemotherapy. Further improvement in image quality can be achieved by using devices with spatial resolution superior to that of 5-in. rectilinear scanner systems, such as large field of view scintillation cameras or the Anger tomographic scanner (Figure 2) (see Chapter 2). The improvement in image quality attainable through these measures is dramatic.

CLINICAL APPLICATION: THE "PREDICTIVE VALUE" IN SELECTED POPULATIONS

Before one can intelligently apply ^{67}Ga scanning to the solution of clinical problems, one must know the predictive value (10) of the test. The predictive value of a positive test (PV pos) has been defined as the percentage of times a patient with a positive test will, in fact, be diseased. It may be calculated as follows:

$$PV\ pos = \frac{\text{number of diseased patients with positive tests}}{\text{total number of patients with positive test}} \times 100.$$

The predictive value of a negative test (PV neg) has been defined as the percentage of times a patient with a negative test will, in fact, be free of disease. It may be calculated as follows:

$$PV\ neg = \frac{\text{number of normal patients with negative test}}{\text{total number of patients with negative test}} \times 100.$$

Of all of the ways in which the "accuracy" of a diagnostic test can be expressed, the PV pos and the PV neg are the parameters that are most meaningful to a clinician. He cannot use test results rationally unless he has some idea of what the chances are that a patient with a positive test has disease and that a patient with a negative test does not have disease.

The PV pos and PV neg cannot be determined directly from the sensitivity and FPR alone. One must also know the prevalence of disease in the population examined, that is, the probability that disease is present in a given patient (or at a given anatomic site) before the test is performed (known as the prior probability of disease being present). Given this prior probability, the sensitivity and FPR, the PV pos and the PV neg can be easily calculated by means of Bayes' theorem (see Appendix A).

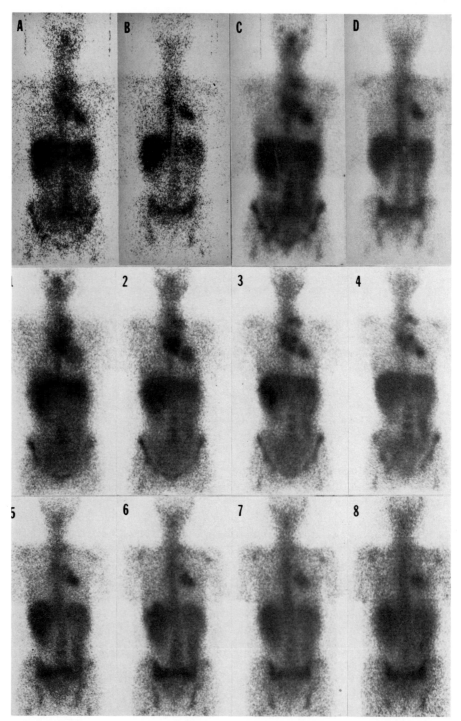

Figure 1. Scanning one photopeak after administration of 3 mCi of ⁶⁷Ga citrate results in poor image quality due to low count density. Image quality will improve dramatically if the count density is increased by use of more than one photopeak and by raising the administered dose of ⁶⁷Ga. These images are of a patient with Hodgkin's disease in the left supraclavicular region, the mediastinum,

For example, let us suppose that we are examining an untreated patient with nodular sclerosing Hodgkin's disease whose only known site of disease is high in the right cervical region. Assuming no constitutional symptoms, the probability of occult abdominal disease is less than 0.1 (i.e., 10%) (11). With a high-resolution scanning device and a high dose (about 10 mCi) of ^{67}Ga, it is reasonable to expect the sensitivity of the scan for abdominal disease sites to be at least 50%, with an FPR of 5% or less (Table 2). In fact, the sensitivity with newer techniques could easily be as high as 70% for abdominal disease sites, with an FPR of 5%, although this possibility has yet to be proven. If we assume a sensitivity of 50%, an FPR of 5%, and a prior probability of 0.1, the PV pos is 53% and the PV neg is 94% (see Table 3 and Appendix A).

Suppose, on the other hand, that we are dealing with a patient with Hodgkin's disease of mixed cellularity whose only known site of disease is in the left supraclavicular region. Assuming no constitutional symptoms, the probability of occult abdominal disease is about 0.5 (i.e., 50%) (11). In this case, the PV pos is 91%, whereas the PV neg is only 66%. Note that, regardless of the outcome of the ^{67}Ga scan, the probability of occult disease in the abdomen will be relatively high.

GALLIUM-67 SCANNING DURING VARIOUS PHASES OF MANAGEMENT OF PATIENTS WITH MALIGNANT LYMPHOMA

Gallium-67 scanning may be applied to the evaluation of patients with malignant lymphoma before a histologic diagnosis is made, during initial staging, and during follow-up evaluation after therapy.

Gallium-67 Scanning Prior to Histologic Diagnosis of Lymphoma

A diagnosis of lymphoma can never be made by means of ^{67}Ga scanning alone, because ^{67}Ga localizes in all types of pathologic tissue (Figure 3). Its usefulness, therefore, is very limited prior to definitive diagnosis by histoligic examination of biopsied tissue. Occasionally, ^{67}Ga scanning might be used to identify possible sites for biopsy when suspicion of lymphoma exists without enlargement of easily accessible lymph nodes.

---

and the hilum and parenchyma of the left lung. The three rectilinear scans (two conventional, one tomographic) were all performed on the same day, 96 hours after intravenous administration of 10 mCi of ^{67}Ga citrate. The scans in the top row were made with a dual-probe 5-in. scanner. The first set of scans (A and B) were obtained by use of the 300 keV photopeak and scanning at 750 cm/min. The maximum count density (80 counts/cm^2 over the liver) is about what one would expect to obtain when scanning that photopeak at the usual speed (250 cm/min) after administration of only 3.3 mCi (0.043 mCi/kg) of ^{67}Ga. In the second set of scans (C and D), the maximum count density was increased to 800 counts/cm^2 by scanning the 185, 300, and 394 keV photopeaks simultaneously in a single 250 keV "wide window." At 250 cm/min, the scan took 50 minutes to complete. The superior image quality due to high count density is typical of "high-dose" (10 mCi) ^{67}Ga scans. The superior spatial resolution of the Anger tomographic scanner (1–4, upper probe; 5–8, lower probe) results in further improvement in image quality. (Maximum count density is 600 counts/cm^2 in this case, because only the 185 keV photopeak was scanned.) Notice that the mediastinal disease is resolved into three separate masses. The definition of the left supraclavicular lesion is clearly superior to that in any of the conventional rectilinear scans.

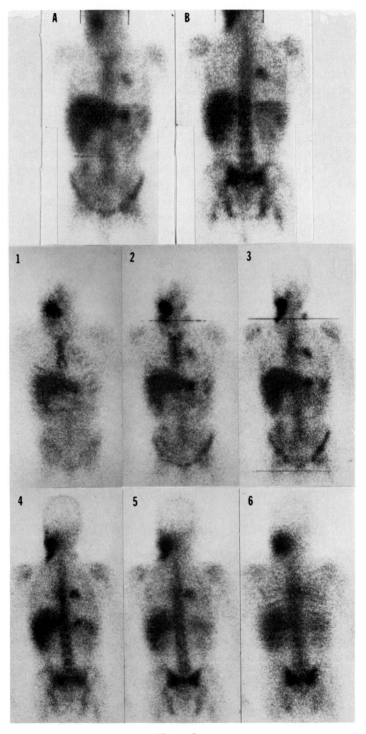

Figure 2.

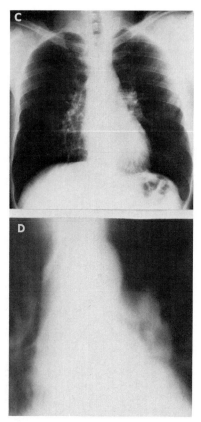

Figure 2, continued.

Figure 2. A 29-year-old male with Hodgkin's disease limited to the right neck (stage I) by clinical evaluation prior to ^{67}Ga scanning. Anterior and posterior views (A and B) made with a dual-probe 5-in. rectilinear scanner demonstrate left hilar disease, not initially appreciated on routine chest roentgenogram (C) but confirmed later by roentgenographic tomography (D). Tomographic ^{67}Ga imaging demonstrates additional disease in left supraclavicular and celiac regions, best seen in anterior planes (scans 1–3). Note tomography shows that celiac disease is deep to left lobe of liver, because it is best seen in deep plane (scan 3). At laparotomy, gross disease was not found; celiac axis node biopsies, directed by ^{67}Ga scan findings, were positive. On sequential posterior planes (scans 4–6), note definition of ribs (scan 6), posterior vertebral structures (scan 5), and vertebral bodies (scan 4). This case clearly demonstrates the superior image quality due to superior spatial resolution of the Anger multiplane tomographic scanner in planes away from the geometric focal plane of the collimator.

TABLE 3 PREDICTIVE VALUE OF POSITIVE AND NEGATIVE TESTS VERSUS
PRIOR PROBABILITY OF DISEASE BEING PRESENT

	Prior Probability of Disease Being Present	PV pos (%)	PV neg (%)
Sensitivity = 50%	0.5	91	66
FPR = 5%	0.1	53	94
Sensitivity = 70%	0.5	93	76
FPR = 5%	0.1	61	97

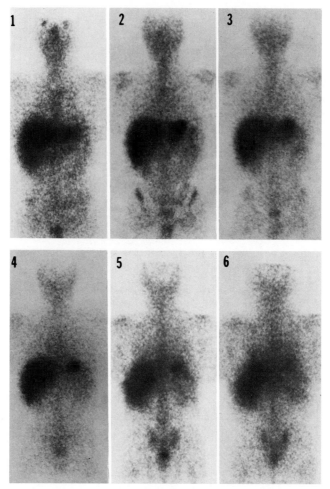

Figure 3.   Gallium-67 uptake is not specific. This 35-year-old male underwent extensive workup for possible recurrence of lymphoma when routine outpatient serum copper determination became elevated after a 5-year disease-free interval. Entire workup, including repeated gastrointestinal studies, proved normal, except for the ^{67}Ga study. Selected tomographic planes from anterior (scan 1) through midplane (scans 3 and 4) to posterior (scan 6) clearly associate the abnormal ^{67}Ga uptake with lesser curvature and fundus of stomach. A benign perforated gastric ulcer was found at laparotomy.

Gallium-67 Scanning During Initial Staging of Patients with Malignant Lymphoma

Accurate knowledge of the extent of malignant lymphoma is crucial in the planning of therapy. Hence, untreated patients with lymphoma are frequently extensively investigated, undergoing numerous procedures, including a careful history and physical examination, radiographic examination of the chest, ^{67}Ga scanning of the entire body above midthigh, lymphangiography, bone marrow biopsy, needle biopsy of the liver, extensive examination of blood and urine, and staging laparotomy (11).

The extent to which ⁶⁷Ga scanning contributes to staging and, ultimately, to management varies with the patient and the clinical problem in question. This variability can be illustrated by the two patients previously cited as examples. Both patients might be candidates for radiation therapy, the extent of which could be influenced by the distribution of disease. If it were known that lymphoma was present in nodal groups above and below the diaphragm, total nodal radiation therapy would be given. If no infradiaphragmatic disease were present, radiation fields could be reduced, provided that constitutional symptoms or other indications for total nodal irradiation were not present. Because of the importance of accurate staging to the planning of therapy, staging laparotomy might be considered for both patients. In the case of the first patient, ⁶⁷Ga could properly influence a decision of whether to operate. Because the prior probability of disease is low (less than 0.1), a negative scan would support a decision to avoid laparotomy (PV neg = 94%), whereas a positive scan would support a decision to operate (PV pos = 53%). For the second patient, however, ⁶⁷Ga scanning would not influence the decision, because the probability of abdominal disease would be relatively high, regardless of the outcome of the scan.

A preoperative ⁶⁷Ga scan may, nonetheless, be helpful in the second patient's case. If positive in the abdomen, it might help guide the surgeon during the staging laparotomy, especialy if a positive site is not easily accessible (e.g., retrogastric lymph nodes) or if the surgeon is not inclined to compulsively sample all major lymph node sites. Occasionally, a ⁶⁷Ga scan will indicate the presence of stage-IV disease by demonstrating lesions in bone or other unsuspected extranodal sites (Figure 4). A positive biopsy from the identified region would, then, render a laparotomy unnecessary.

There are other situations in which ⁶⁷Ga scanning is very useful during initial staging. Patients may refuse to undergo staging laparotomy or laparotomy may be contraindicated because of cardiac or other disease. Gallium-67 scanning and lymphangiography will, then, be the best way of assessing the status of potential abdominal disease sites. (At this writing, the role of computed tomographic scanning and ultrasound in the detection of abdominal lymphoma is uncertain.)

Gallium-67 Scanning After Therapy

Gallium-67 is extremely useful for following the course of a patient's disease after therapy, because it is one of the simplest, least invasive ways of doing so. Serial lymphangiography and staging laparotomy are, of course, much less practical. A positive ⁶⁷Ga scan may be the first or only objective evidence of the persistence or recurrence of treated disease (5) (Figures 5–7). Gallium scanning may be used to distinguish widening of the mediastinum (detected by radiography) due to postirradiation fibrosis from that due to recurrent tumor (12).

It has been suggested that a change in the degree of uptake of ⁶⁷Ga at known disease sites may be used as a quantitative index of the response of tumor to therapy (12). However, it has been pointed out that ⁶⁷Ga uptake may be decreased during or shortly after therapy that is not effective in terms of controlling disease (13). It is generally believed that a positive scan is more reliable than a negative scan after therapy (13).

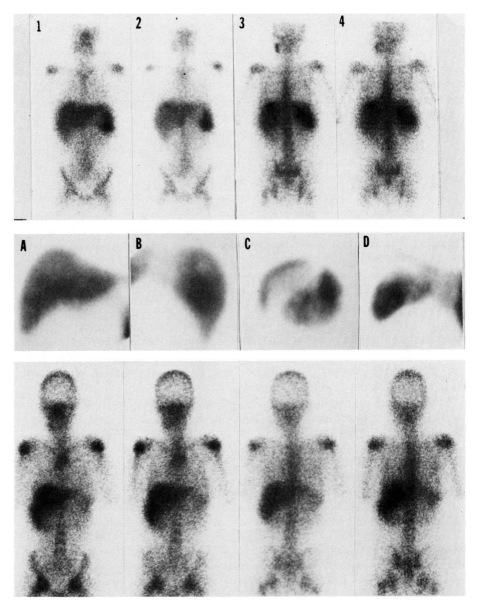

Figure 4. A 12-year-old male with histiocytic lymphoma clinically limited to high posterior right neck was found on ^{67}Ga tomographic scanning (scans 1–4) to have additional disease below the diaphragm. A solitary lesion is apparent in dome of the liver on posterior planes (scans 3 and 4), and more extensive abnormality is seen in anterior aspect of the spleen (scans 1 and 2). Disease was confirmed by ^{99m}Tc-sulfur colloid imaging with discrete lesion on posterior view of liver (B) and multiple coalescing lesions in the spleen on left lateral view (C). Repeat ^{67}Ga scanning (bottom row) 14 months later demonstrates response to chemotherapy.

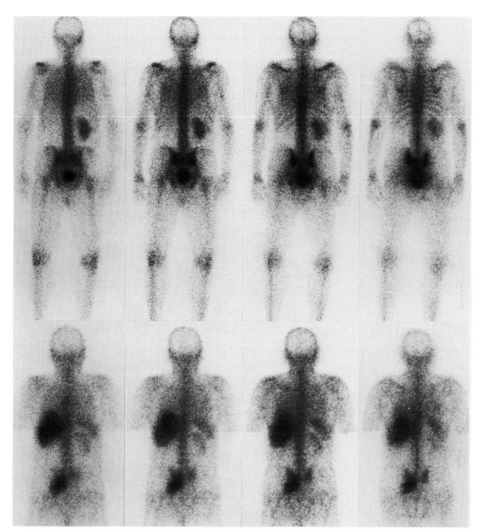

Figure 5. A 62-year-old male with histiocytic lymphoma, who had a previously normal ^{67}Ga scan during a previous period of remission, later developed progressively severe pain radiating down the right leg. Bone scanning (top row), although demonstrating absence of right kidney, failed to indicate the cause of this patient's pain. Selected planes (bottom row) from tomographic ^{67}Ga imagining clearly define disease situated immediately anterior and inferior to the right side of the sacrum, accounting for the pain on the basis of direct involvement of lumbosacral nerve plexus.

CONCLUSIONS

We have attempted to show that ^{67}Ga scanning can be useful in the management of malignant lymphoma, provided that its limitations are kept in mind. One must take into account the apparent variation of lesion detectability with tumor histology and anatomic location. One must always be aware of the nonspecificity of ^{67}Ga scanning. If substantial uncertainty exists regarding the cause of an abnormal focus of activity, and if this uncertainty has significant clinical import,

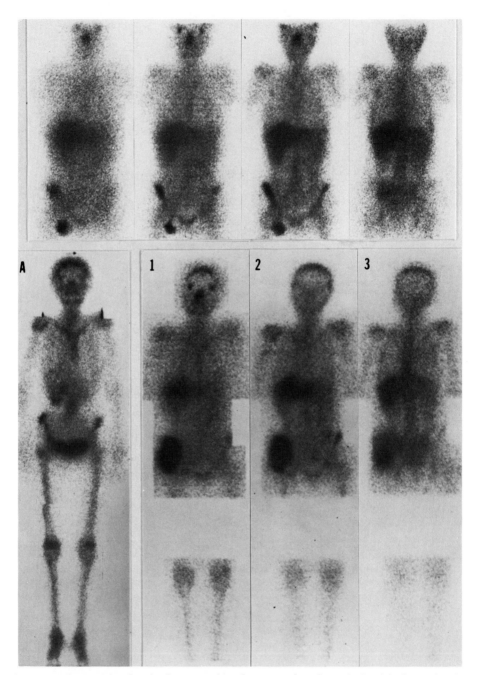

Figure 6.   Nine months after the demonstration of recurrent lymphoma in the right femoral region (selected tomographic planes shown in top row) and treatment with local radiation therapy, this 50-year-old female returned with pain in the right leg. After normal bone imaging (A), extensive local disease infiltrating soft tissues around right side of the pelvis was demonstrated by ^{67}Ga tomographic scanning (scans 1–3). This soft-tissue disease was not apparent on physical examination.

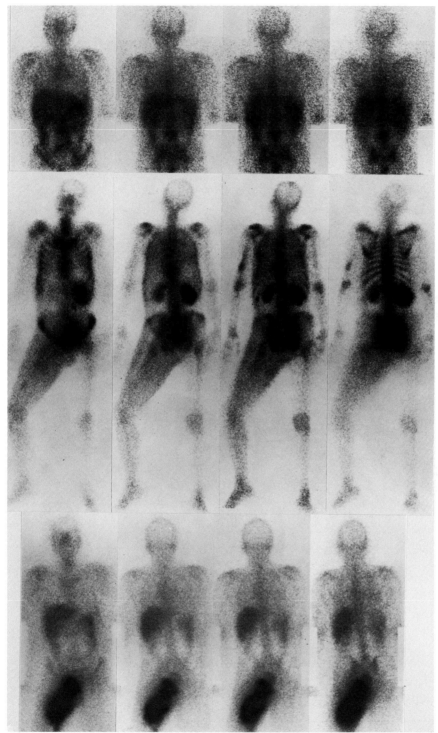

Figure 7.   A 53-year-old female with known lymphocytic lymphoma presented with back pain; tomographic ^{67}Ga scanning (top row) demonstrated disease in the fourth lumbar vertebra. After treatment and a subsequent symptom-free interval, the patient developed a painful swollen right lower extremity with palpable disease above the inguinal ligament. In addition to right leg edema,

histologic examination should be undertaken. It will be found that ^{67}Ga scanning is most useful in following patients after therapy but that it has definite application during the initial staging process.

Finally, when one examines data from series published as of this writing regarding the accuracy of ^{67}Ga scanning in patients with malignant lymphoma, one should realize that the methods used for imaging in these series result in relatively poor image quality. Dramatic improvement can be attained easily through the use of new instrumentation and high doses of ^{67}Ga citrate.

Appendix A

The probability of disease being present, given a positive or negative test, may be determined from Bayes' theorem (14), provided that the true-positive rate (TPR) or sensitivity, the false-positive rate (FPR), and the prior probability of disease being present are known. The probability of disease being present if a test is positive, expressed as a percent, has been termed the "predictive value of a positive test" (PV pos) (10). The probability of disease being absent given a negative test, expressed as a percent, has been termed the "predictive value of a negative test" (PV neg) (10).

$$PV\ pos\ =\ \frac{TPR\ \times\ p(D+)}{TPR\ \times\ p(D+)\ +\ FPR\ \times\ p(D-)}\ \times\ 100, \tag{1}$$

$$PV\ neg\ =\ \frac{TNR\ \times\ p(D-)}{TNR\ \times\ p(D-)\ +\ FNR\ \times\ p(D+)}\ \times\ 100, \tag{2}$$

where:

PV pos = predictive value of a positive test
     = (probability of disease, given a positive test) $\times$ 100,
PV neg = predictive value of a negative test
     = (probability of no disease, given a negative test) $\times$ 100,

$$TPR\ =\ \frac{number\ of\ abnormal\ patients\ or\ sites\ with\ positive\ tests}{total\ number\ of\ abnormal\ patients\ or\ sites}\ \times\ 100,$$

the bone scan (center row) suggested bladder displacement, a poorly functioning obstructed right kidney, and delayed drainage of the left kidney; no direct osseous involvement was apparent. Tomographic ^{67}Ga scanning (bottom row) demonstrated the palpable iliac disease but also revealed extensive infiltration of soft tissue of the upper thigh, unsuspected on physical examination.

Appendix A, Continued

$$\text{FPR} = \frac{\text{number of normal patients or sites with positive tests}}{\text{total number of normal patients or sites}} \times 100,$$

FNR = false negative rate = (100 − TPR),

TNR = true negative rate = (100 − FPR; the TNR has been called the "specificity" of a test),

$p(D+)$ = prior probability of disease being present
 = fraction of abnormal patients or sites in the population being examined,

$p(D-)$ = prior probability of disease being absent
 = $[1-p(D+)]$.

Appendix B

The data reported by Johnston et al. (6) and Greenlaw et al. (7) do not allow direct calculation of their false-positive rate (FPR). However, an estimate of their FPR may be made as follows:

From Appendix A,

$$\text{PV pos} = \frac{\text{TRP} \times p(D+)}{\text{TPR} \times p(D+) + \text{FPR} \times p(D-)} \times 100. \tag{1}$$

Johnston et al. report that eight of 169 biopsied sites positive on scan were histologically negative. Hence, PV pos = 161/169 = 0.95. Their TPR for biopsied sites was 65%. Assuming that $p(D+) = 0.5$, substituting into Equation 1 and solving for FPR, we find that FPR = 3.4%.

If we assume that $p(D+)$ is less than 0.5, the FPR will be less than 3.4%. If $p(D+)$ is as high as 0.7 (very unlikely in their series), the FPR increases to 7.5%. Similar estimates can be made from the data of Greenlaw et al.

REFERENCES

1. Turner DA, Pinsky SM, Gottschalk A, et al: The use of ^{67}Ga scanning in the staging of Hodgkin's disease. *Radiology* **103**:97, 1972.

2. Hoffer PB, Turner DA, Gottschalk A, et al: Whole body radiogallium scanning for staging of Hodgkins disease and other lymphomas. *Nat Cancer Inst Monogr* **36**:277, 1973.

3. Turner DA, Gottschalk A, Hoffer PB, et al: Gallium-67 scanning in the staging of Hodgkin's disease, in Medical Radioisotope Scintigraphy 1972, Vol II, Proceedings of the International Atomic Energy Agency, Vienna, 1973.

4.   Bakshi S, Bender MA: Use of gallium-67 scanning in the management of lymphoma. *J Surg Oncol* **5**:539, 1973.

5.   Henkin RE, Polcyn RE, Quinn JL III: Scanning treated Hodgkin's disease with ^{67}Ga citrate. *Radiology* **110**:151, 1974.

6.   Johnston G, Buena RS, Teates CD, et al: ^{67}Ga-citrate imaging in untreated Hodgkin's disease: preliminary report of cooperative group. *J Nucl Med* **15**:399, 1974.

7.   Greenlaw RH, Weinstein MB, Brill AB, et al: ^{67}Ga-citrate imaging in untreated lymphoma: preliminary report of cooperative group. *J Nucl Med* **15**:404, 1974.

8.   Levi JA, O'Connell MJ, Murphy WL, et al: Role of ^{67}Gallium citrate scanning in the management of non-Hodgkin's lymphoma. *Cancer* **36**:1690, 1975.

9.   Peckham MJ: Value of radiogallium scanning in Hodgkin's disease. *Nat Cancer Inst Monogr* **36**:287, 1973.

10. Vecchio TJ: Predictive value of a single diagnostic test in unselected populations. *N Engl J Med* **274**:1171, 1966.

11. Kadin ME, Glatstein E, Dorfman RF: Clinicopathologic studies of 117 untreated patients subjected to laparotomy for the staging of Hodgkin's disease. *Cancer* **27**:1277, 1971.

12. Patterson AHG, McCready VR: The current status of gallium 67 scanning [Abstract]. *Brit J Radiol* **48**:944, 1975.

13. Andrews GA, Edwards CL: Tumor scanning with gallium-67. *JAMA* **233**:1000, 1975.

14. Green D, Swets JA: Signal Detection Theory and Psychophysics, Reprint with corrections, Robert E. Krieger, Huntington, N.Y., 1974, pp. 14–15.

8
Lung Carcinoma

Carlos Bekerman, M.D.

Clinical Staff
Division of Nuclear Medicine
Michael Reese Hospital and Medical Center

Assistant Professor of Radiology and Medicine
University of Chicago
Pritzker School of Medicine

Chicago, Illinois

Lung carcinoma is the most insidious and commonly lethal of all neoplasms; it is also the most common form of cancer in males. The average survival time after diagnosis is less than 6 months, with a 5-year survival barely approaching 10%. The emphasis in the development of new diagnostic methods has been earlier diagnosis of the disease and better definition of its extent (1–4). Gallium-67 (^{67}Ga) uptake in lung carcinoma was first described by Edwards and Hayes in their original reports of ^{67}Ga uptake in tumors (5,6). Gallium-67 scanning has subsequently become an increasingly widely used method of defining the extent of disease.

Increased uptake of ^{67}Ga in thoracic tumors is easily identified, because radionuclide uptake in normal lung parenchyma is low and activity in the spine, sternum, scapulae, and breast can usually be easily distinguished from tumor uptake (7,8). Positive ^{67}Ga scans are reported to occur in from 64 to 100% of patients with lung carcinoma (9,10) (Figure 1). In a review of results from numerous institutions, Hayes and Edwards (11) reported 194 positive ^{67}Ga scans (85%) in a group of 228 patients with lung carcinoma, including both primary and metastatic lesions. In a more recent review by Larson et al. (12) of a total of 280 reported cases of lung carcinoma, the incidence of positive scans was also 85%. The diagnostic value of ^{67}Ga scintigraphy in patients with lung carcinoma was also assessed by Muhe (13), who found the scans to be more accurate than sputum cytology and bronchoscopy.

The percentage of false-negative ^{67}Ga scans in patients with lung carcinoma ranges from the 22% reported by Hjelms and Dyrbye (14) to 0% reported by Ito et al. (10). The causes for false-negative results are multiple. Among these causes are:

1 Size of the lesion. The majority of lesions not detected on scan are below the limit of resolution of the scanning system (1.5–2 cm) (15).
2. Location of the lesion. Tumor uptake is difficult to detect in right lower lobe lesions, where accumulation of gallium in the liver can mask the activity of the tumor (14).
3. Degeneration and necrosis of the tumor (16).
4. Associated pathology, such as hydrothorax overlying the tumor (Figure 2) or a focus of chronic interstitial pneumonitis surrounding a small carcinoma (17).
5. Administration of cytostatic drugs immediately before the scan (18).

Benign lung lesions may also take up ^{67}Ga (19). Fortunately, many of these lesions (acute infections, sarcoidosis, active tuberculosis) can be distinguished from tumor by means of clinical, laboratory, and radiographic studies. Moreover, not all such benign lesions take up ^{67}Ga. In a group of 55 patients with lesions suspicious of primary carcinoma, DeMeester et al. (20) found that the eight patients with benign lesions all had a negative scan. The histologic diagnoses of those lesions were focal necrosis (two patients), chronic nonspecific granuloma (four patients), hamartoma (one patient), and vascular malformation (one patient).

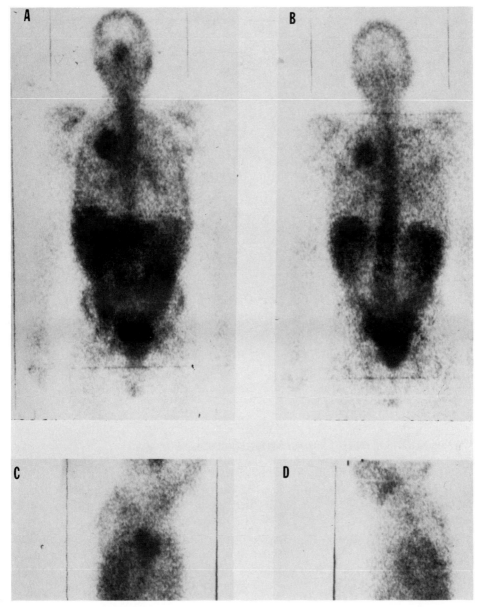

Figure 1. Gallium-67 citrate scan; anterior (A), posterior (B), and lateral (C and D) views of a patient with adenocarcinoma in right upper lobe. Hilar and mediastinal areas are normal.

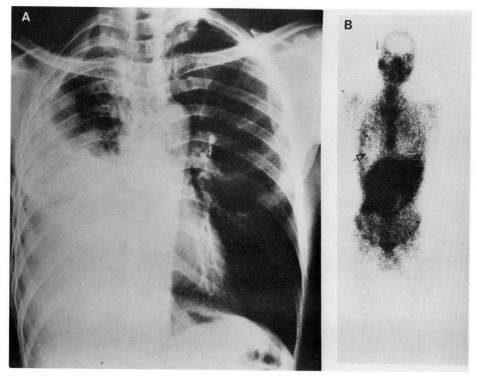

Figure 2.   Chest radiograph (A) and ^{67}Ga citrate scan (B) of a patient with adenocarcinoma of right lower lobe. Area devoid of activity on right hemithorax in the ^{67}Ga scan (arrow) is due to hydrothorax overlying the primary tumor.

CORRELATION OF DETECTABILITY WITH TUMOR HISTOLOGY

According to the classification system of the World Health Organization, 92% of all lung tumors fall into the following histologic categories: epidermoid carcinoma (42%), small-cell anaplastic carcinoma (18%), adenocarcinoma (10%), and large-cell carcinoma (22%) (21). The remaining 8% of tumors include combined epidermoid and adenocarcinomas, carcinoids, bronchial gland tumors, sarcomas, mesotheliomas, melanomas, and otherwise unclassified tumors (22).

Based on histologic examination of a small series (13 cases) of lung tumors, Higasi and Nakayama (23) found the greatest uptake of radionuclide in undifferentiated carcinomas, less in squamous cell tumors, and least in adenocarcinomas. These qualitative results were corroborated by Hjelms and Dyrbye (24), who developed a "relative affinity" ratio to measure relative ^{67}Ga uptake in specimens of normal lung and lung tumor tissue in 31 patients with primary tumors. Their results showed the uptake of ^{67}Ga to be higher in anaplastic and epidermoid tumors than in normal lung tissue (average $R = 3.0$ and 2.8, respectively), while the uptake in bronchogenic adenocarcinomas appeared to be the same as in normal lung tissue (average $R = 1.0$).

In a semiquantitative evaluation, Van der Schoot et al. (25) graded the uptake in the lung lesions by comparing their ^{67}Ga count rate with that of the liver and with a corresponding area of supposedly normal contralateral lung. No relationship between the intensity of tumor uptake and histologic cell type was found.

In a much larger study conducted by an interinstitutional cooperative group (15), the percentage of positive scans according to cell type was 85% for squamous cell well-differentiated tumors, 81% for squamous cell undifferentiated large-cell tumors, 73% for adenocarcinomas, and 70% for small-cell tumors. It was concluded that although there was a slight preponderance of abnormal scans in the squamous cell groups, the other two groups were relatively small compared with the former and that the differences may have been more apparent than real.

Thus most, but not all, of the currently available clinical data indicate that all histologic types of pulmonary carcinoma are associated with a relatively high affinity for [67]Ga.

CORRELATION BETWEEN UPTAKE AND TUMOR SIZE

The most recent and complete classification for bronchial carcinoma is the TNM system (American Joint Committee for Cancer Staging and End Results Reporting) (Table 1). In this system, T designates the primary tumor, N denotes the regional lymph nodes, and M represents distant metastases; the different subgroups (T0, T1, T2, and T3) within the TNM systems have been precisely defined. There is a definite correlation between size of the primary lesion and prognosis. The survival rate is highest for patients with T1 lesions (less than 3 cm in diameter) (26).

DeLand et al. (15) compared the ^{67}Ga scan results with lesion size determined by radiologic or pathologic measurements. Ninety percent of lesions greater than 3 cm in diameter (T2 and T3) were detected on the scan. However, only 43% of primary lesions 2 cm or less in diameter were seen. In a more recent study of 47 patients with histologically confirmed lung carcinoma, the scan was positive in 75% of patients with lesions less than 3 cm in diameter (T1), in 93% of patients with T2 tumors (> 3 cm), and in 97% of patients with T3 lesions (17). Differences in scanning techniques may explain the differences between the results of these two studies. However, no primary lesions smaller than 1.5 cm in diameter were detected in either series. The resolution of routine chest radiographs for primary lung tumor detection is also 1.5 cm (27). Thus, it is still questionable whether the use of gallium scans should be encouraged as a screening test in patients who have only suspicious symptoms (e.g., heavy smokers) but no radiographic evidence for pulmonary disease.

UTILITY AS A FUNCTION OF TUMOR LOCATION

The distinction between peripheral and centrally located tumors is relevant because of its influence on the patient's prognosis. Cellerino et al. (18) and LeRoux and Houlder (28) evaluated the use of ^{67}Ga scans in patients with peripheral lung tumors. The main conventional methods of diagnosis (bronchoscopy, sputum cytology, prescalene node biopsy, mediastinoscopy) very often fail to establish the diagnosis of malignancy in peripheral lesions. In the opinion of

TABLE 1   THE TNM SYSTEM AS A BASIS FOR STAGING OF
           LUNG CANCER (American Joint Committee on
           Cancer Staging, 1972)

T = Primary Tumor

T-0   Tumor proved by the presence of malignant cells in secretions but not vis-
       ualized roentgenographically or bronchoscopically.

T-1   A solitary tumor that is 3.0 cm or less in greatest diameter, surrounded by
       lung or visceral pleura, and without evidence of invasion proximal to a
       lobar bronchus at bronchoscopy.

T-2   A tumor more than 3.0 cm in greatest diameter or a tumor of any size
       which, with its associated atelectasis or obstructive pneumonitis, extends to
       the hilar region. At bronchoscopy, the proximal extent of demonstrable
       tumor must be at least 2.0 cm distal to the carina. Any associated atelec-
       tasis or obstructive pneumonitis must involve less than an entire lung, and
       there must be no pleural effusion.

T-3.1 A superior sulcus tumor with direct extrapulmonary extension.

T-3.2 A tumor of any size associated with (a) atelectasis or obstructive pneu-
       monitis of an entire lung and/or (b) with a pleural transudate negative for
       malignant cells and/or (c) invasion of the chest wall.

T-3.3 A tumor of any size (a) associated with a pleural exudate positive or nega-
       tive for malignant cells, or (b) invading the mediastinum, or (c) less than
       2.0 cm distal to the carina.

N = Regional Lymph Nodes

N-0   No demonstrable spread to the lymph nodes.

N-1   Spread to lymph nodes in the ipsilateral hilar region.

N-2.1 Spread to subcarinal lymph nodes and/or the ipsilateral mediastinal lymph
       nodes adjacent to the distal half of the intrathoracic trachea.

N-2.2 Spread to any other mediastinal lymph node.

M = Distant Metastases

M-0   No distant metastasis.

M-1.1 Spread to scalene and/or supraclavicular lymph nodes.

M-1.2 Spread to any other lymph nodes in the cervical area.

M-1.3 Distant metastasis to liver, bone, brain, etc.

Cellerino and associates (18), the drawbacks of conventional methods constitute
the best indication for the use of ^{67}Ga scans. Ninety-four percent of peripheral
tumors in their series demonstrated increased radionuclide uptake, compared to
only about 50% of benign lesions. Moreover, ^{67}Ga uptake was noted in five of 10
patients in whom the preoperative diagnosis was a benign lesion. All five patients
had malignant lesions confirmed at operation.

Ito et al. (29) were able to establish the malignant nature of hilar masses by
combining ^{67}Ga scintigraphy with perfusion and inhalation scans in 18 cases of
centrally located bronchogenic carcinomas.

DETECTION OF MEDIASTINAL INVOLVEMENT

Evaluation of the mediastinum and hilae is essential for prediction of operability
and for prognosis in patients with lung carcinoma. Many procedures have been
advocated for lymph node assessment. These procedures include comparison of

serial chest x-rays, overpenetrated erect posteroanterior radiographs, shallow right and left anterior oblique radiographs, fluoroscopy, contrast esophagraphy, tomography, contrast studies of the mediastinal vascular structures, and mediastinoscopy. Though all of these methods are useful, none is ideal and some are invasive.

In an early study by Langhammer et al. (30), a site by site analysis of 25 positive ^{67}Ga scans in patients with lung carcinoma demonstrated multiple intrathoracic foci of tumor that had not been revealed by radiography. Siemsen et al. (31) reported that the gallium scan revealed unequivocal mediastinal involvement that had been questionable or not recognized on radiographic studies in 35 of 124 patients with lung tumors. DeLand et al. (15) documented 80% sensitivity for the ^{67}Ga scan in evaluation of 139 lymph node sites in the chest, axillae, and neck classified as proven, apparent, or suspected of harboring metastatic lesions. The sensitivity was somewhat lower for histologically confirmed sites (72%).

Comparison of the results of ^{67}Ga scans for the mediastinum with mediastinoscopy of 55 patients with chest radiograph suspicious for primary lung carcinoma was performed by Bekerman et al. (17). These results are presented in Table 2 (see also Figures 3 & 4). Although the 82% accuracy found for the ^{67}Ga is less than the 89% accuracy reported for mediastinoscopy (32), the scan is a noninvasive procedure, whereas mediastinoscopy is associated with a small but significant incidence of complications (32). Furthermore, the scan may complement mediastinoscopy, improving accuracy by directing the surgeon's attention to regions that are positive on the ^{67}Ga scan and might otherwise be overlooked.

It is sometimes difficult to distinguish between activity in mediastinal lymph nodes and normal gallium uptake in the sternum and thoracic spine (Figure 5). Blending of activity from the primary pulmonary lesion and the sternum may also make it difficult to evaluate the mediastinal lymph node area. The use of lateral scans, dual-isotope subtraction methods, and tomographic scanning devices such as the Anger multiplane tomographic scanner, are all helpful in alleviating this problem to some extent (17,25,33–35).

DETECTION OF HILAR INVOLVEMENT

Despite the numerous radiologic procedures available, there is no good method for evaluation of the hilar nodes other than an exploratory thoracotomy. De-Meester et al. (20) correlated ^{67}Ga scan findings with histologic examination of

TABLE 2   EVALUATION OF "HIGH-COUNT" [67]Ga SCAN
FOR MEDIASTINAL INVOLVEMENT (55 PATIENTS)*

	Histology Positive	Histology Negative
[67]Ga scan positive	18	4
[67]Ga scan negative	6	27
True-positive ratio (sensitivity)	= 0.75	
True-negative ratio (specificity)	= 0.87	
Ratio of correct outcomes to all outcomes (accuracy)	= 0.82	

*From Bekerman et al. (17)

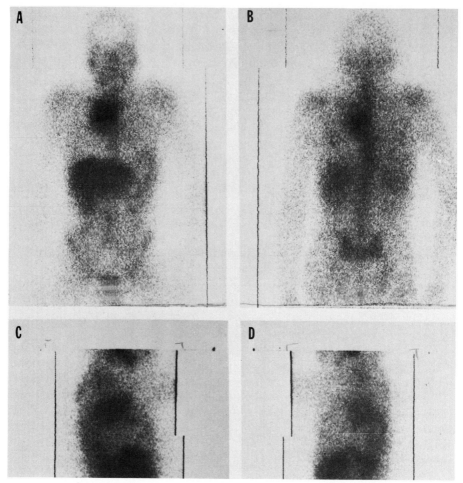

Figure 3.   Gallium-67 citrate scan; anterior (A), posterior (B), and lateral views (C and D) of a patient with adenocarcinoma in right upper lobe with mediastinal involvement.

hilar lymph nodes from 18 patients who underwent surgery (eight pneumonec-tomies and 10 lobectomies). The gallium scans were positive for hilar involve-ment in all 10 patients with proven hilar involvement (Figure 6). However, the scan was also positive for hilar involvement in four of eight patients without histologic evidence of tumor in the hilum. These false-positive results were probably due to overlapping of the primary lesion and hilum (Figure 7).

The ^{67}Ga scan is probably more useful in providing information about the contralateral hilum, because activity from the primary lesion does not interfere with the identification of abnormal lymph nodes in this region (Figure 8). Just as tomographic imaging will probably aid in evaluation of mediastinal lesions, it will also be useful in evaluation of the hilum.

DETECTION OF EXTRATHORACIC TUMOR

Investigation of extrathoracic spread is important in the preoperative evaluation of the patient and for the choice of further radiation or chemotherapy. Unrecognized distant metastases in the liver, bone, brain, or elsewhere are present in about 50% of attempted curative resections (1). At the time of initial treatment, lesions in bone, brain, and other sites were detected on ^{67}Ga scans in about 50% of the patients with lung cancer examined in the cooperative group study (15). Four histologically proven lesions were detected on the scan but were not otherwise suspected; an additional 20 lesions were first detected by the scan and subsequently found to be detectable by other methods (15). The ^{67}Ga scan revealed metastatic involvement in unsuspected areas in 23% of the patients with metastatic carcinoma studied by Littenberg et al. (16). The usefulness of the ^{67}Ga scan in detecting extrathoracic metastases was also evaluated by Bekerman et al. (17). Patients with suspected lung carcinoma had a multiscan evaluation that included brain, liver, bone and ^{67}Ga scans in that order. In 10 patients, the ^{67}Ga scan detected not only the primary lesion but also demonstrated an extrathoracic lesion. Only two of these 10 patients had clinical evidence of extrathoracic tumor at the time of the scan (Table 3). Skeletal lesions were detected in six patients (Figure 9). Only one patient in this group had clinical evidence of bone metastases; five had abnormalities on ^{99m}Tc-EHDP bone scan. Bone biopsies were positive for tumor in all six patients. The uptake of ^{67}Ga by the liver was in-

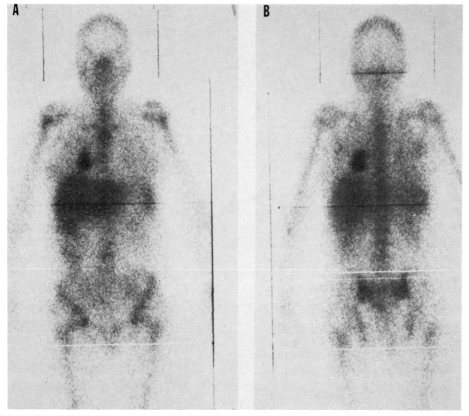

Figure 4.   Gallium-67 citrate scan; anterior (A) and posterior (B) views of a patient with squamous cell carcinoma in right lower lobe. Hilar and mediastinal areas are normal on scan and were found to be normal at mediastinoscopy and thoracotomy.

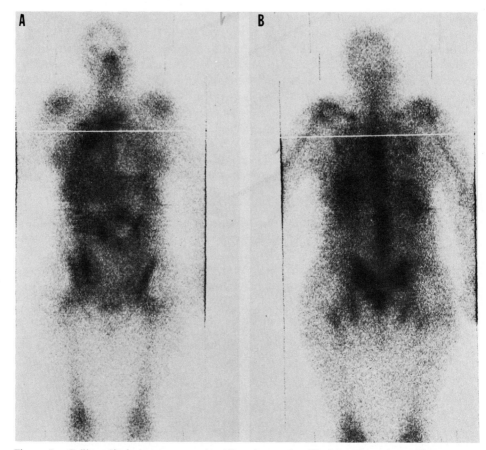

Figure 5.   Gallium-67 citrate scan; anterior (A) and posterior (B) views of a patient with squamous cell carcinoma in right upper and middle lobes. Mediastinoscopy revealed metastatic lymph nodes in upper and anterior mediastinum that had not been identified on the scan because of sternal activity.

homogeneous in one patient and focally increased in the porta hepatis in the other (Figure 10). Neither of these two patients had clinical evidence of metastatic liver disease. The ^{99m}Tc-sulfur colloid scan revealed hepatomegaly in one and a prominent porta hepatis in the other. The liver biopsy was positive for tumor in both patients. In one patient, abnormal ^{67}Ga activity was observed in the left frontal region of the brain (Figure 11). The patient had neurologic symptoms and an abnormal brain scan. Arteriography confirmed a metastatic brain lesion. In another patient, a focal area of increased uptake was noted in the right kidney. A metastasis was demonstrated by renal arteriography.

There are conflicting reports (36,37) about the efficacy of multiorgan scanning in the staging of bronchogenic carcinoma. Perhaps the ^{67}Ga scan could be used to "tailor" further scintigraphic evaluation for extrathoracic metastases in these patients.

PREOPERATIVE STAGING: THE OVERALL PICTURE

The use of the ^{67}Ga scan as an aid to staging patients with lung carcinoma prior to "surgical treatment staging" was evaluated by DeMeester et al. (20). Table 4

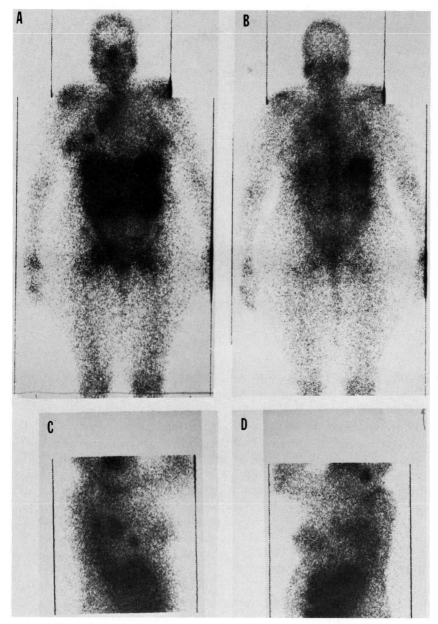

Figure 6.   Gallium-67 citrate scan; anterior (A), posterior (B), and lateral (C and D) views of a patient with small-cell carcinoma of right lower lobe and hilar metastatic lymph nodes. Note the clear separation of the primary lesion and the hilar metastasis.

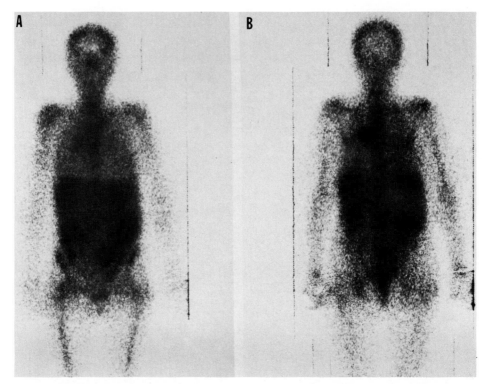

Figure 7.   Gallium-67 citrate scan; anterior (A) and posterior (B) views of a patient with large-cell carcinoma in superior segment of right lower lobe. Due to the location of the primary tumor, it was difficult to evaluate the hilum.

shows the results of a comparative study based on the ^{67}Ga scan and the chest roentgenogram versus the staging after surgical treatment based on histologic examination of the resected surgical specimens. Eighteen patients with lung carcinoma underwent a surgical resection. In only three patients was the staging altered after surgical treatment. Two of the eight patients clinically classified as having stage-II disease were subsequently classified as having stage-III disease. In one patient, there was an extension of the primary tumor into the esophagus; in the other, there were mediastinal lymph node metastases. Five patients were clinically classified as having stage-II disease, and there was no change in the staging after evaluation of the surgical specimen. In one patient, the ^{67}Ga scan was negative, and he was clinically considered to have an occult tumor. The surgical specimen showed a T1 lesion with no metastases to hilar or mediastinal lymph nodes.

In summary, in 15 patients (84%), the pathologic stage remained unchanged; in three cases (16%), a reclassification was made to a more extensive stage; there were no instances of overstaging on the basis of this clinical evaluation. Based on those results, it would seem possible to use the ^{67}Ga scan combined with a chest roentgenogram with a relatively high degree of accuracy in the presurgical staging of patients with suspected lung carcinoma.

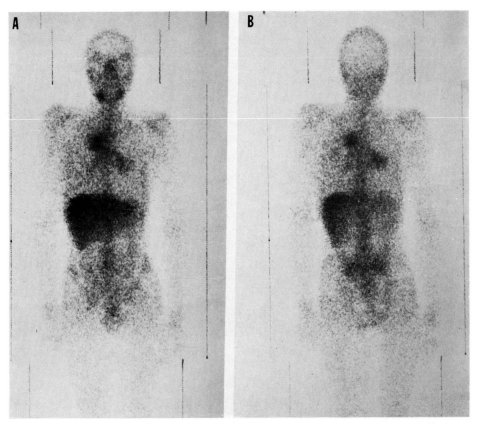

Figure 8.   Gallium-67 citrate scan; anterior (A) and posterior (B) views of a patient with adenocarcinoma in right upper lobe with contralateral hilar involvement confirmed at thoracotomy.

EFFECTS OF TREATMENT ON UPTAKE

Chemotherapy and radiation therapy result in decreased or complete suppression of ^{67}Ga uptake in tumor tissue. In the study reported by Langhammer et al. (30), all patients with lung carcinoma had a negative scan after treatment either

TABLE 3   EXTRATHORACIC SITES OF ^{67}Ga LOCALIZATION*

Number of Patients	Sites of Abnormal ^{67}Ga Localization	Clinical Findings	Results of Other Scans	Confirmed
4	Skeleton	−	^{99m}Tc-EHDP +	Biopsy +
1	Skeleton	−	^{99m}Tc-EHDP −	Biopsy +
1	Skeleton	+	^{99m}Tc-EHDP +	Biopsy +
2	Liver	−	^{99m}Tc-SC +	Biopsy +
1	Brain	+	^{99m}TcO^{4}Na +	Arteriography +
1	Kidney	−	−	Arteriography +

*From Bekerman et al.

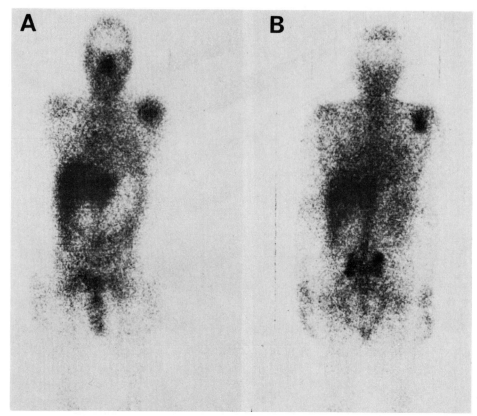

Figure 9.   Gallium-67 citrate scan; anterior (A) and posterior (B) views of a patient with squamous cell carcinoma in right lower lobe and metastatic lesion in left shoulder. Metastatic lesion was confirmed by biopsy.

by chemotherapy or by radiation therapy. Kinoshita et al. (38) reported on 10 patients with pulmonary carcinoma who received a total of 5000–7000 rads delivered within 5–7 weeks. The scans after irradiation were only slightly positive in five cases and were negative in the other five. Some of the lesions that showed no uptake after irradiation had been strongly positive before treatment. There was a good correlation between the change in gallium uptake and the change in tumor size after treatment (determined radiographically).

Kinoshita and associates also attempted to correlate radiation dose with changes in tumor uptake of ^{67}Ga (38). They observed that tumor uptake begins to decrease at about 3000 rads, when compared with pretreatment scans. As previously noted, radiation doses in the 5000–7000-rad range resulted in only slightly positive or negative scans. Kinoshita et al. feel, therefore, that ^{67}Ga scans are useful in guiding radiotherapy for patients with lung tumors (38). If the scan is still slightly positive after 5000 rads, additional radiation should be given. If the scan becomes negative after 4000 rads, radiation therapy may be discontinued at 5000 rads. While the uptake of ^{67}Ga by tumor clearly decreases in proportion to the radiation dose, the exact mechanism that causes this decrease in accumulation of ^{67}Ga is still obscure (23). While some of this effect may be

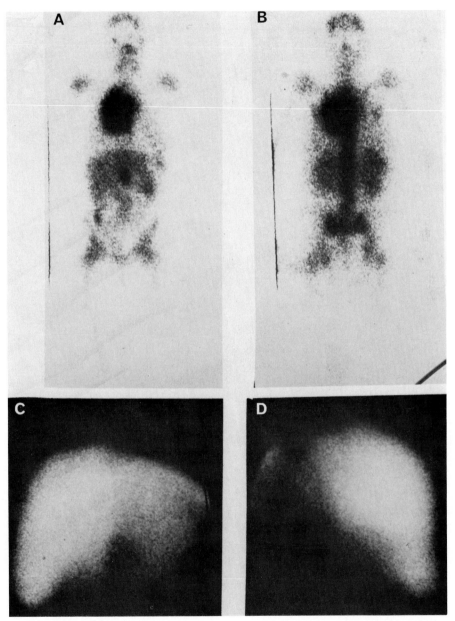

Figure 10. *Top:* Gallium-67 citrate scan; anterior (A) and posterior (B) views of a patient with small-cell carcinoma in right lung with extension into mediastinum. Area of increased uptake is noted in celiac region.

Bottom: ^{99m}Tc-sulfur colloid liver scan; anterior (C) and posterior (D) views of same patient show prominent porta hepatis and umbilical fossa. Metastatic lesion was confirmed by biopsy.

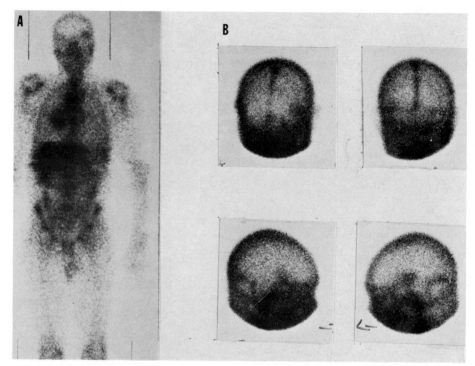

Figure 11.   Gallium-67 citrate scan; anterior view (A) of a patient with squamous cell carcinoma in right middle lobe and mediastinal extension. Area of increased uptake is noted in left frontal region. ^{99m}Tc O^{4}Na brain scan (B) shows area of abnormal uptake in left frontotemporal region. Metastatic lesion as confirmed by arteriography.

TABLE 4   CLINICAL STAGING (CHEST RADIOGRAPH AND ^{67}Ga SCAN) VERSUS POSTSURGICAL TREATMENT STAGING (18 patients)*

		Postsurgical Stage				
		Occult	*I*	*II*	*III*	
	Occult		I			
Clinical (pre-	I		4			
surgical) stage	II			6	2	Clinically un-
	III				5	derstaged: 3
		Clinically overstaged: 0				

*From DeMeester et al.

related to necrosis within the tumor (6), uptake may be suppressed, even when considerable viable tumor remains (12).

Ito and associates speculate that the decrease in uptake after irradiation is due to a combination of decreased volume of viable tumor tissue and suppression of inflammatory processes that accompany neoplastic pulmonary lesions (29). While suppression of gallium uptake in an irradiated tumor does not always indicate eradication of the primary lesion, failure of treatment to suppress uptake is strong evidence that the treatment has not destroyed the primary lesion (16).

It was possible, with the ^{67}Ga scan, to anticipate the appearance of metastatic lesions or recurrences long before they became radiographically visible (23). However, no extensive clinical studies of the use of ^{67}Ga scans to follow patients with lung carcinoma have been reported.

Van der Schoot et al. have reported that some patients scanned immediately after radiation may show slightly increased uptake of ^{67}Ga distributed diffusely in the radiation field (25). No definite explanation exists for this uptake of ^{67}Ga seen shortly after therapy. Van der Schoot et al. (25) postulate that this uptake may occur in the rapidly proliferating connective tissue cells known to be present after radiation treatment. Whatever the explanation, the changes in the distribution of ^{67}Ga citrate in posttreatment scans must be carefully assessed if one is to determine if they represent eradication, incomplete control, recurrence of disease, or benign changes induced by radiation or chemotherapy.

SUMMARY

The ^{67}Ga citrate scan has definite, albeit limited, usefulness in the evaluation of patients with lung cancer.

Detection

A positive scan in a patient with an abnormality on chest radiograph compatible with tumor strongly suggests that the lesion is malignant. However, up to 50% of benign lesions may also accumulate ^{67}Ga. Acute inflammatory lesions are usually responsible for these "false-positive" findings and can often, but not always, be distinguished from tumors on the basis of their radiographic appearance. Unfortunately, a negative scan does not totally exclude the diagnosis of tumor. The scan is therefore useful as a screening test only in patients with radiographic lesions not consistent with inflammatory disease and in whom an invasive workup or exploratory surgery is contraindicated unless the probability of detecting a resectable tumor is high.

The limitations in resolution of the scanning system restrict the possibilities of detecting the lesions before they become radiographically visible. Neither the histologic type nor the location of the tumor seems to affect the probability of detection.

Staging

As a noninvasive procedure, the ^{67}Ga citrate scan complements mediastinoscopy by indicating which lymph nodes should be biopsied. It is also useful in evaluating contralateral hilar node region. The scan also frequently detects clinically unsuspected extrathoracic lesions. It is therefore a useful initial scan procedure in guiding the workup of the patient with known or strongly suspected tumor.

The combination of the ^{67}Ga scan with the chest radiograph could provide the information necessary for presurgical clinical staging in patients with no symptoms that suggest distant metastasis.

Follow-up

Gallium-67 citrate scans may be useful in evaluating the effectiveness of a treatment and the sensitivity of the malignancy to irradiation.

REFERENCES

1. Mountain CF: Keynote address on surgery in the therapy for lung cancer: surgical prospects and priorities for clinical research. *Cancer Chemother Rep Suppl* **4**:19, 1973.

2. Fontana RS: The Mayo lung project for early detection and localization of bronchogenic carcinoma: a status report. *Chest* **57**:511, 1975.

3. Fraser RG, Pare JAP: Diagnosis of Diseases of the Chest, Philadelphia, London, Toronto, Sanders, 1970.

4. Selawry OS, Hensen HH: Lung cancer, in Cancer Medicine, Holland JF, Frei E III (eds), Philadelphia, Lea and Febiger, 1973, p. 1473.

5. Edwards CL, Hayes RL: Tumor scanning with ^{67}Ga-citrate. *J Nucl Med* **10**:103, 1969.

6. Edwards CL, Hayes RL: Scanning malignant neoplasms with gallium 67. *J Amer Med Ass* **212**(7):1182, 1970.

7. Nelson B, Hayes RL, Edwards CL, et al: Distribution of gallium in human tissues after intravenous administration. *J Nucl Med* **13**:92, 1972.

8. Larson SM, Milder MS, Johnston GS: Interpretation of the gallium-67 photoscan. *J Nucl Med* **14**:208, 1973.

9. Grebve SF, Steckenmeser R, Römer M: Radioaktives gallium-^{67}Ga in der nuclear medizinichen Tumor diagnostic. *Münch Med Wochschr* **113**:238, 1971.

10. Ito Y, Okuyama S, Awano T, et al: Diagnostic evaluation of ^{67}Ga scanning in lung cancer and other diseases. *Radiology* **101**:355, 1971.

11. Hayes RL, Edwards CL: New applications of tumor-localizing radiopharmaceuticals, in Medical Radioisotope Scintigraphy, Vienna, International Atomic Energy Agency, 1973.

12. Larson SM, Milder MS, Johnston GS: Tumor-seeking radiopharmaceuticals: gallium-67, in Radiopharmaceuticals, Subramanian G, Rhodes BA, Cooper JF, et al (eds), New York, SNM, 1975, p. 413.

13. Muhe E: Scintigraphic demonstration of bronchial carcinoma using gallium-67 citrate. *Thorax Chir* **10**:440, 1971.

14. Hjelms E., Dyrbye M: ^{67}Ga-scintigraphy in malignant lesions of the lung. *Scand J Resp Diseases* **55**:1, 1974.

15. Deland FH, Sauerbrunn BJL, Boyd C, et al: ^{67}Ga-citrate in untreated primary lung cancer: preliminary report of a cooperative group. *J. Nucl Med* **15**:408, 1974.

16. Littenberg RL, Alazraki NP, Taketa RM, et al: A clinical evaluation of gallium-67 citrate scanning. *Surg Gynecol Obstet* **137**:424, 1973.

17. Bekerman C, DeMeester TR, Skinner DB: The value of "high-count" ^{67}Ga-citrate scans in the staging of lung carcinoma, in Medical Radionuclide Imaging, Vienna, International Atomic Energy Agency, 1977.

18. Cellerino A, Filippi PG, Chiantaretto A, et al: Operative and pathologic survey of 50 cases of peripheral lung tumors scanned with 67 gallium. *Chest* **64**:700, 1973.

19. Van der Schoot JB, Van Marle-van der Goot M, Groen AS, et al: Gallium-67 scintigraphy in benign lung diseases, in Medical Radioisotope Scintigraphy, Vienna, International Atomic Energy Agency, 1973.

20. DeMeester TR, Bekerman C, Joseph JG, et al: Gallium-67 scanning for carcinoma of the lung. *J Thorac Cardiovasc Surg* **72**:699, 1976.

21. Matthews MF: Morphologic classification of bronchogenic carcinoma. *Cancer Chemother Rep* **4**:299, 1973.

22. Kreyberg L: Histological typing of lung tumours. Geneva, World Health Organization.

23. Higasi T, Nakayama Y: Clinical evaluation of ^{67}Ga-citrate scanning. *J Nucl Med* **13**:196, 1972.

24. Hjelms E, Dyrbye M: Uptake of ^{67}Ga in malignant lesions of the lung and lymphatic tissue. *Scand J Resp Diseases* **56**:251, 1975.

25. Van der Schoot JB, Groen AS, de Jong I. Gallium-67 scintigraphy in lung diseases. *Thorax* **27**:543, 1972.

26. Mountain CF, Carr DT, Anderson WA: A system for the clinical staging of lung cancer. *Amer J Roentgenol Radium Ther Nucl Med* **120**:130, 1974.

27. Rigler LB: The earliest roentgenographic sign of carcinoma of the lung. *J Amer Med Ass* **195**:655, 1966.

28. LeRoux BT, Houlder AE: Gallium-67 as a diagnostic tool in the evaluation of peripheral pulmonary lesions. *Thorax* **29**:355, 1974.

29. Ito H, Ishii Y, Sakamato T, et al: Radionuclide studies in bronchogenic carcinoma of the hilum. Scintigraphy and tomography. Their complementary features. *Amer J Roentgenol Radium Ther Nucl Med* **125**:640, 1975.

30. Langhammer H, Hor G, Heidenreich P, et al: Recent advances in tumor scintigraphy, in Medical Radioisotope Scintigraphy, Vienna, International Atomic Energy Agency, 1973.

31. Siemsen JK, Grebe SF, Nicholas Sargent E, et al: Gallium-67 scintigraphy of pulmonary diseases as a complement to radiography. *Radiology* **118**:371, 1976.

32. Jepson O: Mediastinoscopy. Copenhagen, Munksgaard, 1966.

33. Savage PEA, Carmody RG, Highman JH: An evaluation of gallium-67 in the diagnosis of bronchial carcinoma. *Clin Radiol* **27**:202, 1976.

34. Winchell HS, Sanchez PD, Watanabe L, et al: Visualization of tumors in humans using ^{67}Ga-citrate and the Anger whole-body scanner, scintillation camera and tomographic scanner. *J Nucl Med* **11**:459, 1970.

35. McRae J, Anger HO: Clinical results from the multiplane tomographic scanner, in Tomographic Imaging in Nuclear Medicine, Freedman GS (ed), New York, SNM, 1973.

36. Taylor A, Ramsdell JW, Alazraki NP, et al: Efficacy of multiorgan scanning in the staging of epidermoid and adenocarcinoma of the lung. *J Nucl Med* **17**:529, 1976.

37. Operchal JA, Bowen RD, Grove RB: Efficacy of radionuclide procedures in staging of bronchogenic carcinoma. *J Nucl Med* **17**:530, 1976.

38. Kinoshita F, Ushio T, Maekawa A, et al: Scintiscanning of pulmonary diseases with ^{67}Ga-citrate. *J Nucl Med* **15**:227, 1974.

ω

9
Testicular Malignancies

Steven M. Pinsky, M.D.
Director, Division of Nuclear Medicine
Michael Reese Hospital and Medical Center
Associate Professor of Radiology and Medicine
University of Chicago
Pritzker School of Medicine
Chicago, Illinois

Testicular tumor, which usually presents as a solid mass in a testicle, requires surgery with orchiectomy to make the diagnosis. Clearly, this procedure is not desirable if benign disease is present. If gallium were suitable for detection of primary tumors, the number of unnecessary orchiectomies could be reduced. Unfortunately, clinical experience with gallium-67 (^{67}Ga) for detection of primary testicular tumors has been discouraging. Berelowitz and Blake (1) and Littenberg et al. (2) reported single cases of patients with seminoma failing to demonstrate ^{67}Ga uptake in the tumor. Langhammer et al. (3) suggested that gallium is not useful for detection of tumors of the genital system. Only two of six patients in their series showed uptake (one adenocarcinoma of the prostate and one adenocarcinoma of the ovary were successfully detected).

Gallium-67 is useful, however, in the staging of testicular malignancies. Since the treatment of these malignancies is dictated by the specific stage of the disease, meticulous detection and localization of metastases are of the utmost importance. When appropriate noninvasive staging procedures, such as ^{67}Ga scanning, are used, needless radical operations are avoided, and radiotherapy and/or chemotherapy may be instituted more quickly.

A major clinical study was performed at the Walter Reed Army Medical Center in 1973 to determine the value of ^{67}Ga in staging testicular tumors (4,5). The standard workup of a patient with testicular tumor included, in addition to physical examination, chest radiography, lymphangiography, and pathologic examination of the tissue obtained at supraclavicular lymph node biopsy and/or radical retroperitoneal lymphadenectomy. In addition to this workup, a whole-body gallium scan with 3 mCi of ^{67}Ga citrate was performed 48 hours after intravenous injection. Extensive bowel cleansing was performed and was generally quite successful because of the young age of the patients included in the study. The gallium study evaluated abdominal, mediastinal, and supraclavicular lymph node areas for involvement with testicular carcinoma.

Of the first 36 patients studied, there was agreement between the ^{67}Ga scan and biopsy in 33 cases (see Figures 1 & 2). Of the three disparities, two occurred in patients with teratocarcinoma, who had positive lymphangiograms and negative gallium scans but did not undergo surgical evaluation of the retroperitoneal lymph nodes. For the purposes of this study, these cases were considered false negatives. However, these patients have remained well for at least 30 months following staging, and it is believed possible that in these two cases, there was a false-positive lymphangiogram. There was one case of embryonal cell carcinoma that had a completely negative gallium scan, but biopsy was positive for abdominal lymph node involvement. In the majority of cases, the patients had already undergone orchiectomy, and no attempt was made to study primary tumor uptake by gallium.

In all six cases with seminoma (see Table 1), the gallium scan was negative, as was the remainder of the workup. There were 12 patients with embryonal cell carcinoma in this series; six had negative workups and negative gallium scans, and five had positive scans and positive diagnostic workups. There was also one false-negative case among the patients with embryonal cell carcinoma. There were five patients with choriocarcinoma; all had positive scans. Only four of these patients had positive lymphangiograms, but all five were positive on open biopsy. Among the 13 patients with teratocarcinoma, five were negative on both

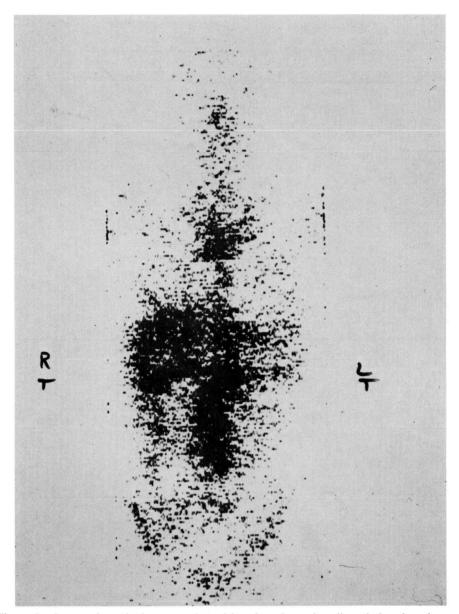

Figure 1.   Increased uptake in retroperitoneal lymph nodes and perihepatic lymph nodes and mediastinum in a patient with testicular cancer. All sites were involved with metastatic tumor.

scan and workup. Two patients were positive on both scan and workup. Four patients had negative scans and positive lymphangiograms. Two of these cases were negative at laparotomy, and the other two were previously mentioned and have not undergone surgery. Two patients with negative scans and questionable lymphangiograms had negative biopsies.

In this study, the gallium scan was found to be more reliable than contrast

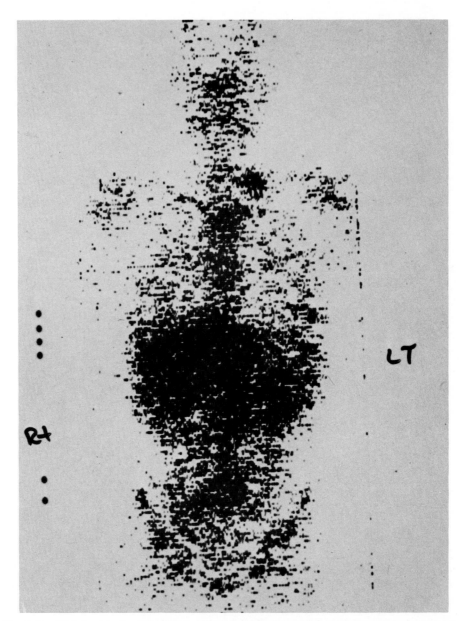

Figure 2.   Metastases to the retroperitoneal lymph node areas and to the left supraclavicular region were demonstrated on the gallium scan of this patient with testicular cancer. Tumor in these areas was proven by biopsy.

lymphangiography when compared to definitive biopsy. Gallium-67 citrate staging in the laparotomy becomes even more valuable when the lymphangiogram cannot be performed due to a variety of reasons, such as allergy to iodinated contrast medium, inadequate equipment, history of severe cardiac or pulmonary disease, previously unsuccessful attempt at lymphangiography, or prior injury to or extensive operations in the lower extremities, abdomen, or pelvis. These contraindications to lymphangiography do not apply to gallium scans. The gal-

TABLE 1   DETECTION OF LYMPH NODE INVOLVEMENT IN TESTICULAR CARCINOMA

	Number of Cases	Scan Results	Workup
Seminoma	6	All negative	All negative
Embryonal cell carcinoma	12	7 negative	6 negative, one positive
		5 positive	5 positive
Choriocarcinoma	5	5 positive	5 positive
Teratocarcinoma	13	11 negative	9 negative
			2 positive by lymphangiogram only
		2 positive	2 positive

lium scan may also be helpful in the not infrequent occurrence of a questionable lymphangiogram.

During the course of this study, one patient with unsuspected supraclavicular metastasis was detected only by the gallium scan; a pulmonary metastasis was detected in another patient prior to visualization by standard chest radiography. The whole-body gallium scan in patients with testicular carcinoma has also been demonstrated to be of use in the follow-up of previously treated disease. Similar results have been shown in patients with Hodgkin's disease who are followed by gallium scan (6). It is important to remember that a positive gallium scan after radiation therapy or chemotherapy is highly suggestive of recurrence; however, a negative gallium scan after radiotherapy or chemotherapy does not rule out recurrence. The posttherapy gallium scan may be of great value, because alternative diagnostic procedures, such as laparotomy or lymphangiography, are usually not employed for follow-up.

The group at Walter Reed Medical Center obtained two interesting gallium scans of the testicles. One in a patient with cystic teratoma showed complete absence of gallium uptake on the side of the cystic lesion. In another case with epididymo-orchitis, definite tumor-like uptake of ^{67}Ga citrate was noted. These cases emphasize that ^{67}Ga may not be taken up in primary testicular tumors but may be taken up in nonmalignant lesions that mimic testicular cancer.

In summary, ^{67}Ga citrate appears to be of no benefit in determining the etiology of testicular masses. It has been shown to be taken up in inflammatory diseases of the testicles and to be absent in several primary testicular tumors. However, once the diagnosis of testicular carcinoma is confirmed, ^{67}Ga citrate seems to play a major role in both the staging of the disease and in the follow-up of patients who have already undergone therapy. A recent clinical study by Paterson and associates (7), performed to evaluate the role of the ^{67}Ga scan in staging seminomas, supports the findings of the original Walter Reed study.

REFERENCES

1. Berelowitz M, Blake KCH ^{67}Gallium in the detection and localization of tumors. *S. Afr Med J* **45**:1351, 1971.

2. Littenberg RL, Alazraki NP, Taketa RM, et al: A clinical evaluation of gallium-67 citrate scanning. *Surg Gynecol Obstet* **137**:424, 1973.

3.   Langhammer H, Glaubitt G, Grebe SF, et al: [67]Ga for tumor scanning. *J Nucl Med* **13**:25, 1972.

4.   Pinsky SM, Bailey TB, Blom J, et al: ^{67}Ga-citrate in the staging of testicular malignancy. *J Nucl Med* **14**:439, 1973.

5.   Bailey TB, Pinsky SM, Mittemeyer BT, et al: A new adjuvant in testis tumor staging: gallium-67 citrate. *J Urol* **110**:307, 1973.

6.   Henkin RE, Polcyn RE, Quinn JF: Scanning treated Hodgkin's disease with ^{67}Ga-citrate. *Radiology* **110**:151, 1974.

7.   Paterson AHG, Peckham MJ, McCready VR: Value of gallium scanning in seminoma of the testis. *Brit Med J* **1**:1118, 1976.

10

Childhood Malignancies

Carlos Bekerman, M.D.

Clinical Staff
Division of Nuclear Medicine
Michael Reese Hospital and Medical Center

Assistant Professor of Radiology and Medicine
University of Chicago
Pritzker School of Medicine

Chicago, Illinois

Cancer is the most common lethal disease in children between the ages of one and 15 years. However, the survival rate of pediatric patients with malignant neoplasias has dramatically improved in recent years. This success is due not only to improved therapeutic approaches (1) but also to the increasing accuracy of defining the anatomic extent of disease at the time of diagnosis, which, in turn, provides a more rational basis for planning of therapy (2,3).

Among the many diagnostic tools now employed in the "staging" process is gallium-67 (^{67}Ga) citrate scanning. This procedure has been used extensively for tumor localization in a broad spectrum of neoplastic diseases in adults. However, there have been very few studies of its use in childhood malignancies (4–11). The results of these studies will be reviewed in this chapter. Emphasis will be placed on both the utility and the limitations of ^{67}Ga scintigraphy in specific types of childhood malignancies.

LYMPHORETICULAR NEOPLASMS

Hodgkin's Disease and Other Lymphomas

The clinical characteristics of Hodgkin's disease and of other lymphomas are considerably different between children and adults. It has been speculated that the juvenile form of Hodgkin's disease is actually a distinct pathologic process (12–17). The juvenile form occurs predominantly in males (91%) and is usually either the nodular sclerosing or the lymphocytic predominant type (16,18). According to Strum and Rappaport (12), these two histologic types have a favorable prognosis.

The diagnosis of juvenile Hodgkin's disease is usually made by surgical biopsy of a cervical lymph node. Asymptomatic adenopathy is the most common presenting sign. Occasionally, the child presents with respiratory symptoms caused by bronchial obstruction due to a mediastinal mass. Less than 30% of children present with systemic symptoms.

Accurate staging of Hodgkin's disease is especially important in children. The disease cannot be cured or controlled unless all sites of involvement are treated. However, both radiation therapy and chemotherapy may have severe effects on growth and development. If the extent of the disease is known precisely prior to treatment, these complications can be minimized. In children, splenectomy is accompanied by the risk of subsequent overwhelming pneumococcal sepsis. Therefore, any noninvasive method that obviates the need for splenectomy is highly desirable.

Chest radiography is useful to detect mediastinal disease. Hematologic studies are of limited value, because the marrow is rarely involved in children in the absence of radiographic bone changes. Lymphangiography in children is difficult to perform and almost as difficult to interpret (19,20).

Although the use of the ^{67}Ga scan in the staging of Hodgkin's disease has been studied extensively (see Chapter 7), very few studies have investigated specifically the juvenile form of the disease.

Gallium scintigraphy was evaluted by Lepanto et al. (6) in seven children with Hodgkin's disease. Of 11 sites known to be involved by tumor, seven were positive on scan. Five of them were located above the diaphragm, and two were intra-abdominal. Two false-negative results occurred in patients with Hodgkin's involvement of celiac and para-aortic lymph nodes. The one false-positive result was due to an area of tumor-free inflammatory lymphadenopathy.

We have studied 13 children with lymphoreticular neoplasms who had a ^{67}Ga scan as part of their initial clinical evaluation (10). Their histologic diagnosis and pathologic stages according to the Ann Arbor classification are presented in Table 1.

Eleven patients underwent a staging laparotomy, which consisted of retroperitoneal lymph node dissection and biopsy, splenectomy, needle biopsy of the right and left lobes of the liver, and a wedge biopsy of the right lobe. A total of 113 sites were evaluated on scan and correlated with the clinical radiologic and histologic findings. Of 31 proven sites of disease, 27 were positive on scan, giving a sensitivity of 87%. This figure is similar to that obtained in larger series composed mostly of adults (21–37). All 82 sites free of disease were negative on scan (specificity = 100%).

The results of this study, evaluated by anatomic area, are shown in Table 2. All mediastinal lesions were positive on scan (Figure 1,B). In two patients, the ^{67}Ga citrate scan was more sensitive than the chest radiograph, revealing lesions that were later confirmed by tomography in one patient and by mediastinoscopy and biopsy in another. These findings confirm the known sensitivity of gallium scintigraphy for detection of mediastinal lesions (34). However, due to the problem of thymic uptake of gallium in children, mediastinal uptake in the thymic region should be confirmed by other studies before being considered due to tumor. Eleven of the 14 histologically positive peripheral lymph nodes in this group of patients were identified on gallium scan, giving a sensitivity of 79% (Figure 1,A).

TABLE 1   HISTOLOGIC DIAGNOSIS AND DISEASE STAGE IN 13 CHILDREN WITH LYMPHORETICULAR NEOPLASMS STUDIED WITH GALLIUM SCANS*

Histologic Diagnosis	Stage	Number of Patients
Hodgkin's disease		
Nodular sclerosing	II	3
Nodular sclerosing	IIE (chest wall)	1
Nodular sclerosing	III (spleen)	3
Nodular sclerosing	IV (lung)	1
Mixed-cell type	I	2
Mixed-cell type	II	1
Malignant lymphomas		
Poorly differentiated lymphocytic	IV (bone marrow, cerebrospinal fluid)	1
Histiocytic lymphoma, diffuse	III (spleen)	1

*From Beckerman et al. (10)

TABLE 2 CORRELATION BETWEEN ^{67}Ga SCAN RESULTS AND NUMBER OF
SITES INVOLVED BY LYMPHORETICULAR NEOPLASMS*

	Mediastinum	Superficial Lymph Nodes	Para-aortic and Iliac Lymph Nodes	Spleen	Liver	Other Areas	Total
Involved sites	10	14	1	4	0	2[†]	31
True positives	10	11	1	3	0	2	27
False positives	0	0	0	0	0	0	0
True negatives	3	40	21	7	11	—	82
False negatives	0	3	0	1	0	0	4

*From Bekerman et al. (10).
[†]The two areas of involvement were chest wall and lung, both of which were confirmed by biopsy.

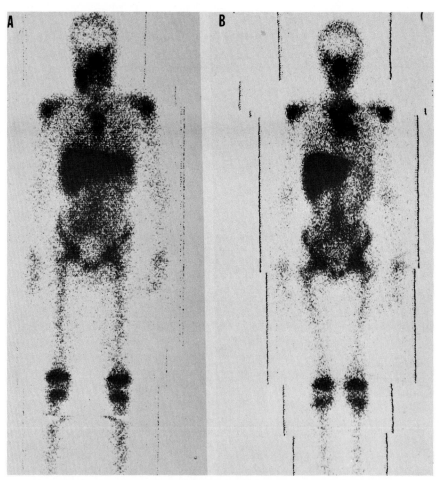

Figure 1. A: Gallium-67 citrate scan (anterior view) in a 9-year-old girl with Hodgkin's disease, nodular sclerosing, PS I-A. Abnormal activity is noted in the right cervical region. The increased activity in the epiphyseal regions is normal in children. B: Gallium-67 citrate scan (anterior view) in a 10-year-old girl with Hodgkin's disease, nodular sclerosing, PS II-A. Abnormal activity is noted in the hilum of the left lung, anterior mediastinum, and right and left supraclavicular fossae.

The intra-abdominal lymph nodes have traditionally been difficult to evaluate by the ^{67}Ga citrate scan in adults because of colonic excretion and accumulation of the radionuclide. This factor may explain, in part, the somewhat low accuracy obtained in the evaluation of the intra-abdominal lymph node groups (32,33,37,38). There were no false-positive or false-negative results in the evaluation of intra-abdominal lymph node sites in our series. The only site involved by lymphoma in the para-aortic iliac lymph nodes was detected by the ^{67}Ga citrate scan. The high accuracy of the gallium scan in the abdomen in children is probably due to the fact that there is less bowel accumulation of radionuclide in children than in adults. Also, very thorough bowel preparation and a triple-window high-count-density imaging technique were used in this study (38,39).

Scintigraphy of the spleen with ^{99m}Tc-sulfur colloid is not a completely reliable indicator of lymphomatous involvement (40). Increased uptake of gallium by the spleen, as compared with the liver, was observed in three of four children with splenic involvement in our study. Although gallium uptake in reactive splenomegaly is seen in adult Hodgkin's disease, we observed no such cases (10). The possibility of assessing splenic involvement in children based on the estimate of gallium uptake deserves further investigation. The gallium-67 scan is less sensitive in the detection of lymphomatous involvement of the liver than conventional colloid scintigraphy.

There are no reports of the use of ^{67}Ga citrate scans to follow children with lymphoreticular neoplasms. However, based on the experience with adults, ^{67}Ga scintigraphy could play a valuable role in measuring the effectiveness of treatment in children with lymphoma (36) (Figure 2).

Despite some limitations, ^{67}Ga scintigraphy is a noninvasive procedure that provides useful information for clinical staging of children with lymphoma. It may be useful as a substitute for lymphangiography, which is difficult to perform on small children. For planning of radiation ports, the ^{67}Ga citrate scan could provide highly useful information on the size and location of lesions. The gallium scan may also be useful to evaluate the effectiveness of treatment and detect early recurrence of disease.

Burkitt's Lymphoma

Among the malignant lymphomas, Burkitt's tumor constitutes a distinct clinicopathologic syndrome. Its excellent response to chemotherapy, the possible participation of host defense mechanisms in tumor regression, and its probable viral etiology have all made this tumor the subject of intensive investigation. Burkitt's lymphoma occurs predominantly in children between the ages of 2 and 14 (peak incidence at 7 years) who live in warm, moist climates. The tumor is characterized histologically by the absence of appreciable cellular differentiation toward either lymphoid or histiocytic cells. More than half of the cases present clinically with maxillar and mandibular involvement. The second most common presentation is as an abdominal tumor. The organs usually involved are the kidneys, ovaries, mesentery, and retroperitoneal tissue. Liver and spleen are less frequently involved. Tumor involvement of peripheral lymph nodes is rare, occurring in only 5% of patients. Involvement of the central nervous system is common. Chemotherapy is usually the treatment of choice. Dramatic remissions often occur. Survival is closely related to the clinical stage. Stages I or II have a good prognosis, with an estimated 2-year survival of 81%. Stage-III tumors have

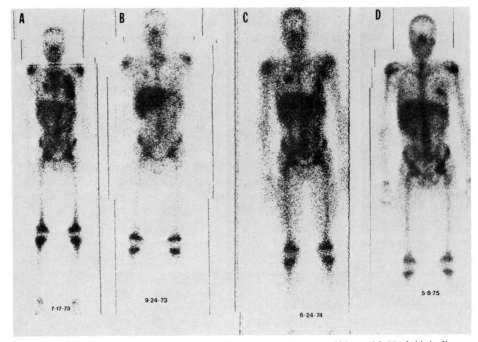

Figure 2.   A: Baseline ^{67}Ga citrate scan (anterior view) in a 14-year-old boy with Hodgkin's disease, nodular sclerosing, PS IV-B (lung). Abnormal uptake is noted in the left lung and right lung hilum (7/17/73). B: Follow-up ^{67}Ga citrate scan after radiation and chemotherapy. The lesion in the left lung has resolved, but activity is still seen in the right lung. A new lesion is also seen in the left supraclavicular fossa. Note the decreased activity in mediastinum and increased salivary uptake, both due to radiation therapy (9/24/73). C: There is now reappearance of left lung abnormality and increase in size of the right hilar mass. The left supraclavicular mass has resolved (6/24/74). D: Gallium-67 citrate scan after chemotherapy reveals resolution of the right hilar mass and residual focus of lymphoma in left lower lobe (5/8/75).

a survival rate of 64% at 2 years. The least favorable prognosis is for stage-IV patients, who have an estimated survival of 52% at one year. Relapse in patients who have been treated assumes different patterns, depending on the duration of the initial remission (41).

An extensive evaluation of ^{67}Ga radionuclide imaging in Burkitt's lymphoma has been conducted by Richman et al. (7). Fourteen American patients were studied in whom the diagnosis of Burkitt's tumor was established by its distinct histologic and cytologic features. Eighteen of the 31 whole-body gallium images performed on these patients were abnormal and showed intense gallium accumulation by the tumor. There was good correlation between the gallium scan findings and the known, or clinically suspected, sites of tumor involvement. The extent of tumor was accurately delineated in all patients. Scans were negative when the patients were examined during complete clinical remission. All children with relapse of Burkitt's lymphoma had positive ^{67}Ga scans.

Soft-tissue Sarcomas

Soft-tissue sarcomas usually present as a mass, which is asymptomatic until it causes pressure against, or traction on, a nerve. The diagnosis is made by histopathologic study of tissue obtained by biopsy. Radiographs of the affected area may demonstrate calcifications within the mass or invasion of bone. Arteriography may reveal the characteristic hypervascularity of these tumors. It will also disclose the relationship between the tumor and neighboring osseous and neurovascular structures. Soft-tissue sarcomas usually metastasize to the lung; therefore, chest radiographs and whole-chest tomograms are useful for both initial evaluation and for follow-up.

Gallium-67 citrate scans in patients with soft-tissue sarcomas were evaluated by Lepanto et al. (6). Of a total of 16 sites known to be involved by tumor, only six were positive on scan. Six of the eight false-negative lesions were bone metastases. The remaining two false-negative lesions were lung metastases. The sensitivity of gallium scan in this study was only 43%. One false-positive region was also recorded.

We have also used gallium scintigraphy as part of the initial evaluation in 11 patients with soft-tissue sarcomas (10). The histologic subtypes were as follows: six rhabdomyosarcomas, two undifferentiated sarcomas, one fibrosarcoma, one neurosarcoma, and one mixed-cell type of sarcoma. Nine of the tumors were located peripherally; four in the extremities and five in the head and neck. The remaining two patients had retroperitoneal tumors (Figure 3). Of a total of 15 sites considered clinically and histologically involved by tumor, 14 were positive on scan. In one patient, a clinically unsuspected metastasis in the left lung hilum was detected by scan and subsequently confirmed at surgery. In two patients, bone metastases documented by radiographic survey and bone scan were also positive on gallium scan. In one of the patients with retroperitoneal tumor, only part of the large mass showed activity, whereas the remaining portion appeared as a "photon-deficient" area (Figure 3,A). This finding was attributed to hemorrhage or necrosis within the large tumor mass (no chemotherapy or radiation had been administered). The one false-negative result occurred in a patient with multiple small lung metastases that were demonstrated on chest radiograph.

Experience with the use of the ^{67}Ga citrate scan as a monitor for therapy in soft-tissue sarcomas is minimal. Mussa et al. (9) and Edeling (11) both reported a total of four patients who had scans after radiation and/or chemotherapy. The scans detected local recurrence of the primary lesion, in addition to regional and distant metastases.

PRIMARY TUMORS OF BONE AND CARTILAGE

Osteosarcoma and Ewing's sarcoma are the most common primary bone tumors in children. The peak incidence for both tumors occurs in the 10–25-year age range, and both are more common in males than in females. Osteosarcoma occurs most commonly in the lower femur; the tibia and humerus are the next most common sites. These three bones account for 85% of all such lesions. Any bone may be involved by Ewing's sarcoma; however, it is most frequently found

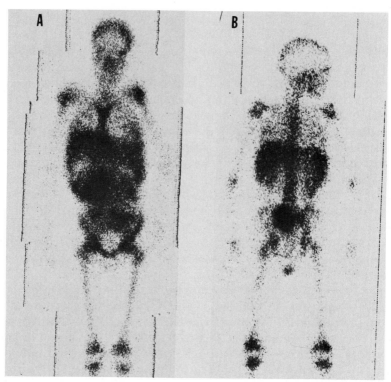

Figure 3.   A: Gallium-67 citrate scan (anterior view) in a 15-year-old boy with a retroperitoneal
soft-tissue sarcoma in the right flank and right lumbar fossa. Uptake is increased only in the bottom
portion of the large mass; the remaining parts of the tumor appear devoid of activity. B: Gallium-67
citrate scan (posterior view) in a 10-year-old boy with an undifferentiated presacral sarcoma with
invasion of the sacrum.

in the femur, pelvis, ribs, tibia, humerus, vertebrae, fibula, and scapula in that
order. Pain, tenderness, and swelling are common accompaniments of these
tumors. They may also be associated with fever and weight loss. The radionuclide bone scan is a sensitive method of detecting both tumors. Histologic examination of biopsy or surgical specimens is required to definitely establish the
diagnosis. Nonetheless, the radiologic appearance frequently suggests the
diagnosis. Osteosarcomas occur in the metaphysis, cause periosteal reaction,
produce either lytic, sclerotic, or mixed patterns of change in involved bone,
and are usually associated with a soft-tissue mass. Ewing's sarcoma occurs most
commonly in the diaphysis or metaphysis; it may also show variable degrees of
patchy, lytic bone destruction. Subperiosteal reactive new bone formation in
Ewing's sarcoma often has a layered, "onion skin" appearance. Extensive longitudinal involvement of the bone may occur, and extension into overlying soft
tissue is common. Angiograms are useful to evaluate the extent of soft-tissue
involvement around the tumor. Clinical laboratory tests generally are not useful in the diagnosis of primary bone tumor, although they may assist in the
differential diagnosis and early diagnosis of recurrence (42).

   Osteosarcomas usually metastasize first to lung and only subsequently to other
organs, including bone (except in cases of local extension). Ewing's sarcoma is

more likely to metastasize to bone early and without pulmonary involvement. McNeil and associates (43) have emphasized the value of the chest x-ray in early detection of metastatic osteosarcoma and of the bone scan for detection of metastatic Ewing's sarcoma.

The gallium-67 citrate scan and other diagnostic modalities were evaluated in patients with primary bone tumors of the Ewing's sarcoma type by Frankel et al. (8). In a combined retrospective and prospective study of 27 patients with biopsy-proved Ewing's sarcoma, radionuclide (^{67}Ga citrate scans and bone scintigraphy with ^{18}F or ^{99m}Tc-polyphosphate), radiographic, and clinical data were correlated.

The diagnosis of a malignant bone tumor was made from the initial radiographic study in 26 of the 27 patients. The one false-negative result occurred because overlying colonic stool repeatedly obscured an iliac lesion. Bone scan was also positive in 26 primary tumors, including the above-mentioned iliac lesion. A tumor of the S-1 vertebra was the only lesion not seen with bone scintigraphy. Fifteen patients had a ^{67}Ga citrate scan at the time of initial evaluation. They all were positive in the region of the primary tumor, including the one case that was false-negative on bone scan (Table 3). As in McNeil's study (43), the bone scan was more sensitive than the radiograph for detecting skeletal metastases. Ninety-two percent of the lesions were detected by bone scintigraphy, whereas the radiographic bone survey detected only 30%. Gallium scintigraphy detected 60% of lesions and was therefore better than radiography but not as good as the bone scan.

A total of 13 extraskeletal metastatic sites were found in this series. In only one of eight lung lesions did the ^{67}Ga scan detect the abnormality prior to chest radiography. The detection data for all extraskeletal sites are summarized in Table 4. Analysis of follow-up scans for the site of previously treated primary tumor revealed that most of the lesions had persistently increased uptake of nuclide on either bone or ^{67}Ga scans (62% of cases). Twenty-four percent of lesions showed decreased uptake, and 13% had normal uptake in the region of the tumor. The roentgenographic studies remained abnormal in all cases.

The authors concluded that ^{67}Ga citrate scintigraphy is more sensitive than radiography for the detection of primary and metastatic skeletal lesions; however, it was less sensitive than the bone scan. Extension of the primary tumor into overlying soft tissues is more easily detected by the ^{67}Ga citrate scan than by bone scan or radiographic studies and therefore aids in the design of the radiation

TABLE 3   CORRELATION OF RESULTS WITH ^{67}Ga STUDIES, SKELETAL SCANS, AND RADIOGRAPHY IN EWING'S SARCOMA*

	[67]Ga Study	Bone Scan	Radiography
Primary	15/15[†]	26/27	26/27
Skeletal metastases	8/13	12/13	4/13
Extraskeletal metastases	4/13	0/13	9/13

*From Frankel et al. (8).
[†] All values are number positive per total number detected.

TABLE 4   GALLIUM STUDIES COMPARED WITH RADIOGRAPHY IN ABILITY TO
DETECT EXTRASKELETAL METASTASES TO VARIOUS SITES IN
PATIENTS WITH EWING'S SARCOMA*

Organ	Total number of Metastases	Number of [67]Ga Positive	Number of X-ray Positive
Lung	8	1	7
Mediastinum	1	1	0
Pleura	1	1	0
Abdominal lymph nodes	2	1	1
Spinal cord	1	0	1

*From Frankel et al. (8).

ports. The poor sensitivity of the ^{67}Ga citrate scan for detecting extraskeletal
metastatic sites (mainly the lungs) indicates that it cannot be used as a substitute
for the radiographic study of the chest. Gallium-67 scintigraphy, however, as a
single diagnostic procedure, permits the evaluation of possible tumor involvement in any organ. Anatomic areas particularly difficult to assess radiographically, such as mediastinum and retroperitoneum, are probably better evaluated
by means of the ^{67}Ga scan. The main use of ^{67}Ga citrate scans in patients with
Ewing's sarcoma is an adjunctive procedure for the detection of early subclinical
metastases.

NEUROBLASTOMAS

Neuroblastomas originate from neural crest elements and are composed of im-
mature neural cells. The tumor possesses a specific antigen capable of stimulating
antibody formation, which may suppress the growth of neuroblastoma cells in
tissue cultures. Neuroblastoma usually occurs in neonates and young children. It
occurs only rarely after the age of 14. Clinically, these children frequently present with an abdominal mass that may be asymptomatic. Neuroblastomas metastasize widely and unpredictably; in infants and young children, liver metastases
are common. Intravenous pyelography is helpful to differentiate neuroblastoma
from Wilms' tumor of the kidney. Neuroblastomas usually displace but do not
invade the renal parenchyma. Neuroblastomas synthesize catecholamines, and
their metabolites can often be detected in the urine.

   Gallium-67 scintigraphy was evaluated in three patients with proven neuroblastoma in 12 clinically known metastatic sites by Lepanto et al. (6). The primary
tumors were positive on scan, whereas all of the metastatic sites were negative.
Nine were skeletal metastases, and three were soft-tissue lesions. Littenberg et al.
(22) observed only a 50% incidence of ^{67}Ga uptake in neuroblastomas. We have
observed a similar low incidence of ^{67}Ga uptake in a group of eight children with
neuroblastoma (10). Twenty-three proven sites of disease were evaluated; of
those, only 10 were positive on scan. Most of the negative sites were skeletal
metastases. Based on the ^{67}Ga citrate scan results, the patients were divided into

two categories: a "positive uptake" group and a "negative uptake" group. The positive uptake group consisted of three patients in whom not only the primary tumor but also all documented metastases showed marked and avid uptake of radionuclide (Figure 4); the negative uptake group consisted of five patients in whom the primary and secondary sites showed normal or less ("photon-deficient") activity than did the surrounding normal tissues (Figure 5). No clear relationship was found between the degree of ^{67}Ga citrate uptake and cellular differentiation or amount of lymphocytic infiltration of the tumors. None of the patients in the negative uptake group received chemotherapeutic drugs or radiation therapy before the scan, nor did they have clinical evidence for complications, such as hemorrhage or necrosis within the tumor mass. The two groups of patients had a completely different clinical course that could not be correlated to the initial staging. All of the patients in the positive uptake group did very poorly, whereas four children in the negative uptake group were in clinical remission 30 months after the diagnosis of neuroblastoma had been established.

The rather poor results obtained in all series indicate that ^{67}Ga citrate is not

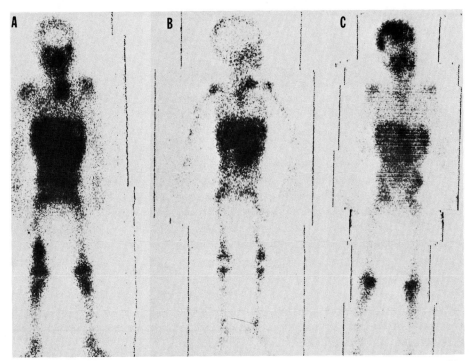

Figure 4.   A: Gallium-67 citrate scan (anterior view) in a 4-year-old boy with stage-IV neuroblastoma. Abnormal uptake is noted in the left supraclavicular fossa, mediastinum, and left paratracheal region. Below the diaphragm, increased activity is noted in the left paraspinal and midperiaortic areas. A bone metastasis is also visible in the right distal femur. B: Gallium-67 citrate scan (anterior view) in a 5-year-old boy with stage-IV neuroblastoma. Activity in left retroperitoneal mass and left supraclavicular lymph node is noted. C: Gallium-67 citrate scan (anterior view) in a 5-year-old boy with stage-IV neuroblastoma. Uptake in left para-aortic mass and in skull metastases is noted.

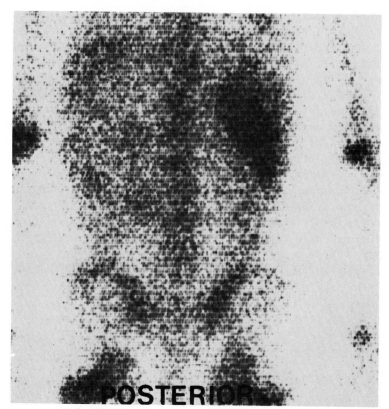

Figure 5.   Gallium-67 citrate scan (posterior view of abdomen) in a 12-year-old boy with stage-IV neuroblastoma. Photo-deficient area is noted in the right upper quadrant, corresponding to location of the tumor.

useful for the staging or follow-up evaluation of patients with neuroblastoma. Most of the primary lesions are positive on scan; it is interesting to note that practically all of the false-negative results corresponded to skeletal metastases. We have no clear explanation for the failure of ^{67}Ga uptake in the osseous lesions. The significance of the negative uptake and its relation with the survival rate is unclear and deserves further evaluation.

OTHER TUMORS

The limited information available concerning the use of ^{67}Ga in patients with Wilms' tumor and other, less common pediatric malignancies suggests that gallium imaging is not useful for staging or follow-up.

SUMMARY

Gallium scanning is useful in the staging and follow-up of pediatric patients with Hodgkin's disease and Burkitt's lymphoma. It has more limited value in the evaluation of soft-tissue sarcomas, osteosarcoma, and Ewing's sarcoma. It is probably not useful in the evaluation of patients with neuroblastoma or Wilms' tumor.

Gallium may be taken up in the normal thymus and in the epiphyses in children, and these sites should not be mistaken for tumor.

REFERENCES

1. Holleb AI: Children and cancer [Editorial]. *Ca–A Cancer J Clinicians* **26**(2):128, 1976.
2. National Office of Vital Statistics: Vital Statistics of the United States, 1959. Washington, D.C., United States Public Health Service, Department of Health, Education, and Welfare.
3. Murphy ML: Curability of cancer in children. *Cancer* **22**:779, 1968.
4. Edwards CL, Hayes RL: Tumor scanning with ^{67}Ga-citrate. *J Nucl Med* **10**:103, 1969.
5. Silberstein EB: Reviews: Cancer diagnosis. The role of tumor imaging radiopharmaceuticals. *Amer J Med* **60**:226, 1976.
6. Lepanto PB, Rosenstock J, Littman P, et al: Gallium-67 scans in children with solid tumors. *Amer J Roentgenol Radium Ther Nucl Med* **126**:179, 1976.
7. Richman SD, Appelbaum F, Levenson SM, et al: ^{67}Ga-radionuclide imaging in Burkitt's lymphoma. *Radiology* **117**:639, 1975.
8. Frankel RS, Jones AE, Cohen JA, et al: Clinical correlations of ^{67}Ga and skeletal whole-body radionuclide studies with radiography in Ewing's sarcoma. *Radiology* **110**:597, 1974.
9. Mussa GC, Madon E, Martini-Mauri M, et al: La ricerca di lesioni neoplastiche con radiogallio nei bambini. *Minerva Ped* **27**:1137, 1975.
10. Bekerman C, Port RB, Pang E, et al: Scintigraphic evaluation of childhood malignancies by ^{67}Ga-citrate-scintigraphy. Unpublished data.
11. Edeling CJ: Tumor imaging in children. *Cancer* **38**:921, 1976.
12. Strum SB, Rappaport H: Hodgkin's disease in the first decade of life. *Pediatrics* **45**:748, 1970.
13. Hays DM: The staging of Hodgkin's disease in children reviewed. *Cancer* **35**:973, 1975.
14. Jenkin RDT, Brown TC, Peters MV, et al: Hodgkin's disease in children. A retrospective analysis: 1958–73. *Cancer* **35**:979, 1975.
15. Butler JJ: Hodgkin's disease in children, in Neoplasia in Childhood, Chicago, Year Book Medical, 1969, pp. 267–279.
16. Evans HE, Nyhan WL: Hodgkin's disease in children. *Johns Hopkins Med J* **114**:237, 1964.
17. Kelly F: Hodgkin's disease in children. *Amer J Roentgenol Radium Ther Nucl Med* **95**:48, 1965.
18. Patchefsky AS, Brodovsky H, Southard M, et al: Hodgkin's disease—a clinical and pathologic study of 225 cases. *Cancer* **32**:150, 1973.
19. Kadin ME, Glatstein E, Dorfman RF: Clinicopathologic studies of 117 untreated patients subjected to laparotomy for the staging of Hodgkin's disease. *Cancer* **27**:1277, 1971.
20. Nuland SB, Prosnitz LR: Exploratory laparotomy and splenectomy in Hodgkin's disease. *Amer J Surg* **125**:399, 1973.
21. Edwards CL, Hayes RL: Scanning malignant neoplasms with gallium-67. *J Amer Med Ass* **212**:1182, 1970.
22. Littenberg RL, Alazraki NP, Taketa RM, et al: A clinical evaluation of gallium-67 citrate scanning. *Surg Gynecol Obstet* **137**:424, 1973.
23. Winchell HS, Sanchez PD, Watanabe CK, et al: Visualization of tumors in humans using ^{67}Ga-citrate and the Anger whole-body scanner scintillation camera and tomographic scanner. *J Nucl Med* **11**:459, 1970.
24. Langhammer H, Glaubitt G, Grebe SF, et al: ^{67}Ga for tumor scanning. *J Nucl Med* **13**:25, 1972.
25. Ito T, Okuyama S, Awano T, et al: Diagnostic evaluation of ^{67}Ga scanning of lung cancer and other diseases. *Radiology* **101**:355, 1971.
26. Manfredi OL, Quinones JD, Bartok SP: Tumor detection with gallium-67 citrate, in Medical Radioisotope Scintigraphy, Vol 2, Vienna, International Atomic Energy Agency, 1973, p. 583.

27. Berelowitz M, Blake KCH: ^{67}Gallium in the detection and localization of tumors. *S Afr Med J* **45**:1351, 1971.

28. Lavender JP, Barker JR, Chaudhri MA: Gallium-67 citrate scanning in neoplastic and inflammatory lesions. *Brit J Radiol* **44**:361, 1971.

29. Silberstein EG, Kornblut A, Shumrick DA, et al: ^{67}Ga as a diagnostic agent for the detection of head and neck tumors and lymphoma. *Radiology* **110**:605, 1974.

30. Sims JC, Tauxe WN, Goel WS, et al: ^{67}Ga-citrate imaging. *J Nucl Med Tech* **1**:20, 1974.

31. Jones AE, Koslow M, Johnston G, et al: ^{67}Ga-citrate scintigraphy of brain tumors. *Radiology* **105**:603, 1972.

32. Turner DA, Pinsky SM, Gottschalk MD, et al: The use of ^{67}Ga scanning in the staging of Hodgkin's disease. *Radiology* **103**:97, 1972.

33. Johnston G, Benua RS, Teates DD, et al: ^{67}Ga-citrate imaging in untreated Hodgkin's disease: preliminary report of cooperative group. *J Nucl Med* **15**:399, 1974.

34. Kay DN, McCready VR: Clinical isotope scanning using ^{67}Ga-citrate in the management of Hodgkin's disease. *Brit J Radiol* **45**:437, 1972.

35. Bakshi S, Bender MA: Uses of gallium-67 scanning in the management of lymphoma. *J Surg Oncol* **5**:539, 1973.

36. Henkin RE, Polcyn RE, Quinn JL: Scanning treated Hodgkin's disease with ^{67}Ga-citrate. *Radiology* **110**:151, 1974.

37. Greenlaw RH, Weinstein MD, Brill AB, et al: ^{67}Ga-citrate imaging in untreated malignant lymphoma: preliminary report of cooperative group. *J Nucl Med* **15**:404, 1974.

38. Hoffer PB, Turner DA, Gottschalk A, et al: Whole body radiogallium scanning for staging of Hodgkin's disease and other lymphomas. *Nat Cancer Inst Monogr* **36**:277, 1973.

39. Turner DA, Gottschalk A, Hoffer PB, et al: Gallium-67 scanning in the staging of Hodgkin's disease, in Medical Radioisotope Scintigraphy, Vol II, Vienna, International Atomic Energy Agency, 1973, pp. 615–630.

40. Milder MS, Larson SM, Bagley CM Jr, et al: Liver-spleen scan in Hodgkin's disease. *Cancer* **31**:826, 1973.

41. Ziegler JL: Burkitt's tumor, in Cancer Medicine, Holland JF, Frei E (eds), Philadelphia, Lea and Febiger, 1973, pp. 1321–1330.

42. Sutow WW, Martin RG: Bone and cartilagenous tumors, in Cancer Medicine, Holland JF, Frei E (eds), Philadelphia, 1973, pp. 1863–1879.

43. McNeil BJ, Cassady RJ, Geiser CF, et al: Fluorine-18 bone scintigraphy in children with osteosarcoma or Ewing's sarcoma. *Radiology* **109**:627, 1973.

11

Other Malignancies in Which Gallium-67 Is Useful: Hepatoma, Melanoma, and Leukemia

Carlos Bekerman, M.D.

Clinical Staff
Division of Nuclear Medicine
Michael Reese Hospital and Medical Center

Assistant Professor of Radiology and Medicine
Unive rsity of Chicago
Pritzker School of Medicine

Chicago, Illinois

Paul B. Hoffer, M.D.

Professor of Diagnostic Radiology
Director, Section of Nuclear Medicine
Yale University School of Medicine
New Haven, Connecticut

MELANOMA

Malignant melanoma is a tumor that derives from pigment-producing melano-
cytes. More than 90% of melanomas originate in the skin, with 50–70% arising in
a preexisting nevus. The most frequent sites of metastases are the adjacent skin
and regional lymph nodes (1). Surgical resection of the primary tumor in the
absence of detectable metastasis is curative in more than 90% of patients. However, distant and clinically unsuspected tumor spread is not uncommon.

A comprehensive evaluation of the value of the gallium scan in patients with
malignant melanoma was performed by Milder et al. (2). The study consisted of
a retrospective and prospective evaluation of 44 consecutive patients with tumor
thought to be surgically curable. A total of 48 gallium scans were reviewed. In 22
of the patients, a direct assay of gallium-67 (^{67}Ga) activity was performed on
selected samples of tumor and adjacent normal tissue obtained at surgery 72
hours after administration of radiopharmaceutical.

Fifty-four percent of grossly involved or pathologically proven sites with
malignant melanoma were detected by scan. When sites clinically suspected to be
involved by tumor but not pathologically studied were evaluated, the scan results
were almost the same (52%). The ^{67}Ga scan was normal in 98% of sites in which
melanoma was excluded by gross or microscopic pathologic examination. The
results were similar when sites with normal clinical and radiologic evaluation but
with no pathologic study were evaluated. The false-positive rate was not more
than 2%. Some of the false-positive sites were the result of recent surgery. The
remaining sites, however, may have represented the earliest evidence for metastatic disease.

The incidence of missed lesions was 45%. The size of the tumor mass greatly
influenced the sensitivity of the scan results. Tumors larger than 2 cm were
detected by ^{67}Ga scanning in 75% of cases, whereas those 2 cm or less in size were
found only 11% of the time. The location of the lesion also influenced the
detection rate. All bone lesions were accurately detected; lymph node metastases, which constituted the most frequent sites of involvement, were visualized
in 60% of the known cases. Lung, brain, and liver involvement was correctly
diagnosed in over 60% (Figure 1). Skin and subcutaneous tumors were detected
less than 50% of the time. Lesions in other organs, such as gastrointestinal tract,
kidneys, and adrenals, were visualized in 45% of the cases (Figure 2). No ocular
melanomas were studied in this group of patients.

In vitro studies demonstrated a strong affinity of melanoma for ^{67}Ga. Involved lymph nodes and subcutaneous masses had the highest tumor to background ratios. Despite these high ratios, some of the lesions were not visualized
on scan, probably due to their small size. The autoradiographic studies
confirmed the presence of activity within the tumor. Gallium-67 did not appear
to be bound to melanin and was taken up equally by melanotic and amelanotic
tumors.

Thirty-six consecutive patients with proven malignant melanoma in stages III
and IV were studied with ^{67}Ga citrate scans during their initial work-up and at
subsequent intervals by Jackson et al. (3). The scan findings were correlated with
other evidence of disease, for example, findings of biopsy, major surgery, autopsy, radiographic examination and/or clinical examination. The overall results
with ^{67}Ga scintigraphy in determining the extent of disease were superior to

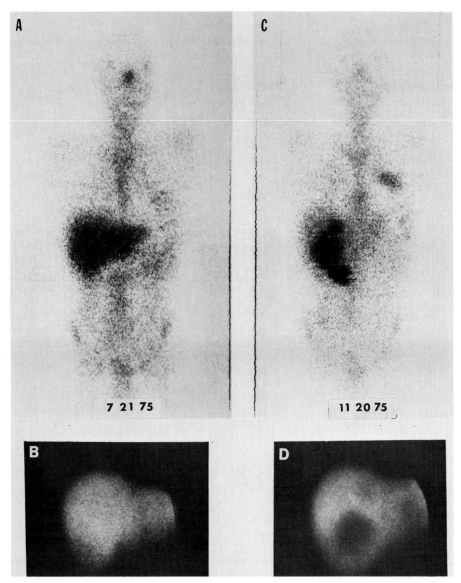

Figure 1. Patient with malignant melanoma resected. The initial postoperative gallium (A) and liver (B) scans were normal. Five months later a gallium scan reveals metastatic lesions in the left lung and in the liver (C). The gallium-positive liver lesions correspond to the new defects seen on the liver scan (D).

those obtained by Milder et al. (2). About 70% of gallium positive regions were histologically confirmed sites of tumor involvement. The histologically confirmed false positive rate was only about 5%. (The other 25% of positive areas were not biopsied.) While Jackson and associates did not provide exact statistics for scan negative regions, they report the incidence of false negatives to be low. They also compared scan findings to patient survival. The life expectancy of patients with a normal scan was longer than that of patients with an abnormal scan (3).

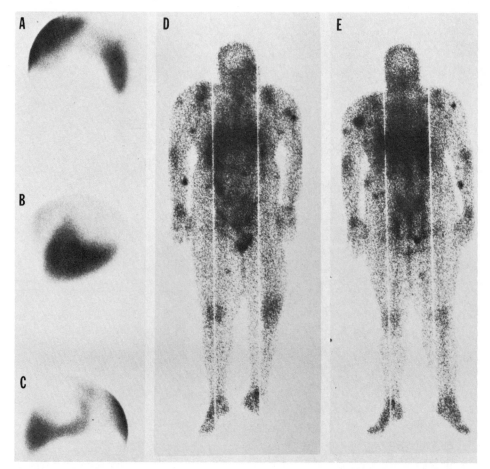

Figure 2.   Patient with suspected recurrent malignant melanoma. Anterior (A), lateral (B) and posterior (C) views of the spleen. (^{99m}Tc sulfur colloid) reveal a large splenic mass. Anterior (D) and posterior (E) views of the gallium scan reveal multiple skin lesions. The large splenic mass shows intense uptake. (Courtesy of E. Nijensohn, M.D. Christ Hospital, Oak Lawn, Illinois.)

In summary, gallium scintigraphy is a useful method for detection of clinically unsuspected metastases from malignant melanoma. A positive scan is highly suggestive of metastatic spread. Unfortunately, a negative scan does not rule out the presence of metastatic disease. A negative gallium scan also has some favorable prognostic significance.

In view of the affinity of melanoma for gallium, the major limitation of the ^{67}Ga scan in detecting metastasis seems to be technical, that is, the inability of most imaging instruments to resolve the small metastatic lesions. The Anger tomoscanner may be particularly useful in overcoming this problem (Figure 5, Chapter 3).

HEPATOMA

Hepatoma is an infrequent primary tumor in America. Predisposing conditions include cirrhosis (either postnecrotic or alcoholic), hemochromatosis, clonarchiasis, Fanconi's anemia, and irradiation. The diagnosis of hepatoma is frequently masked by the preexisting hepatic disease. Jewel (4) reported that only 20% of cases were diagnosed correctly antemortem or preoperatively. The α-fetoprotein assay is a relatively specific test for this disease but may be negative in from 25 to 50% of cases. The ^{99m}Tc-sulfur colloid liver scan is usually abnormal, but the "cold" areas due to hepatoma often cannot be distinguished from cold areas due to the so-called pseudotumors, or regenerative nodules, of cirrhosis. Because most hepatomas occur in patients with cirrhosis, the diagnosis can only rarely be established based on the ^{99m}Tc-sulfur colloid scan alone.

When discussing gallium scanning of hepatic lesions, it is important to define what is meant by the term "increased gallium uptake." The liver normally concentrates a large fraction of the injected dose of ^{67}Ga citrate and is prominent on most gallium images. Uptake in many "gallium-positive" lesions is no greater than uptake in normal liver tissue. Gallium uptake in a hepatic lesion is defined not in relation to gallium uptake elsewhere in the liver but in relation to ^{99m}Tc-sulfur colloid uptake in the same region. A lesion that has decreased ^{99m}Tc-sulfur colloid uptake compared to the remainder of the liver but that exhibits gallium uptake equal to the rest of the liver is considered to have "increased gallium uptake" and be "gallium positive." Therefore, the liver cannot be adequately assessed by the gallium scan without an accompanying ^{99m}Tc-sulfur colloid liver scan. A liver with multiple areas of "increased gallium uptake" may have a perfectly uniform appearance on the gallium scan (Figure 3).

Increased gallium uptake is observed in most hepatomas (5–9) but rarely occurs in the so-called pseudotumors, or regenerative nodules, of cirrhosis.* The gallium scan is therefore useful in distinguishing between these two lesions. The increased uptake of gallium in hepatoma has been confirmed by tissue assay in animals (13). Increased gallium uptake also occurs in most hepatic abscesses, in about 50% of metastatic liver tumors, and in benign hepatic adenomas (14). Therefore, increased gallium uptake is not specific for hepatoma. The reported incidences of increased gallium uptake in hepatoma and in numerous other hepatic lesions are presented in Table 1. Suzuki and associates (5) report that hypervascular hepatomas are more likely to be positive on gallium scan than are hypovascular lesions. Suzuki and coworkers (8) also observed a high detection rate for hepatoma with gallium, even in patients with negative serum α-fetoprotein (AFP) tests. This observation has been disputed by Levin and Kew (9), who detected increased gallium uptake in hepatomas in only six of 12 patients with hepatoma and negative AFP titers.

LEUKEMIA

Gallium scanning has been evaluated on a limited basis as a diagnostic procedure for the care of patients with acute (15) and chronic (16) leukemias. Its chief benefit in acute lymphocytic and acute myelogenous leukemias is its localization in the inflammatory lesions that accompany these diseases. This localization is dependent on an adequate population of leukocytes. In chronic granulocytic

---

*Normal or increased gallium uptake has been reported to occur in regenerating liver tissue in animals after partial hepatectomy (10–12). These findings should not be confused with the clinical observation that the regenerative nodules of cirrhosis do not usually take up gallium.

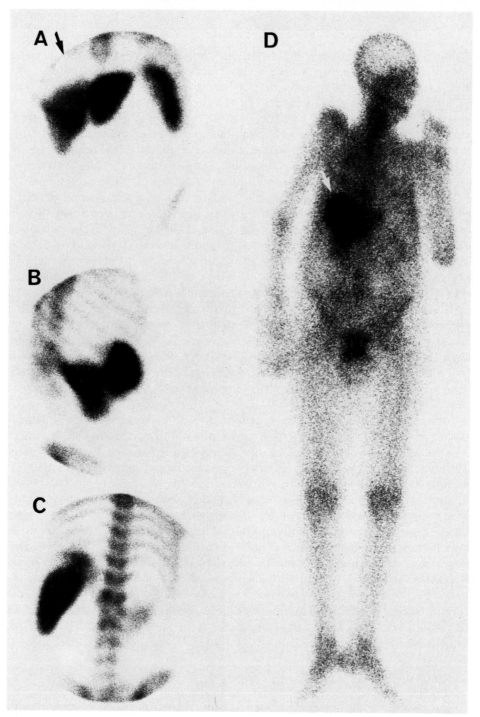

Figure 3.   Anterior, right lateral and posterior projection (A, B and C) of ^{99m}Tc-S-Colloid scan showing a mass lesion in superior and posterior aspect of right hepatic lobe. There is also splenomegaly with increased colloid uptake by spleen and bone marrow. The later findings are typical of parenchymal liver disease. The anterior projection of the gallium scan (D) reveals gallium uptake in the mass (arrow) seen in the colloid scan. The gallium scan itself shows relatively uniform uptake and might be considered "normal" in the absence of the colloid scan. (Courtesy of E. Nijensohn, M.D., Christ Hospital, Oak Lawn, Illinois.)

TABLE 1   INCIDENCE OF ^{67}Ga-POSITIVE LESIONS OF THE LIVER

Series	Total Number of Patients	Hepatoma	Pseudotumor of Cirrhosis	Metastasis
Lomas et al.* (6)	63	12/12†	3/11	13/17
Suzuki et al. (5)	19	7/7		5/11
Hamamoto et al. (7)	29	10/11		7/16
Suzuki et al. (8)	71	26/27		12/39
Levin and Kew (9)	38	26/38		—

*These figures are different from those usually quoted and are based on the criteria described in the text.
†All values are number positive per total number of patients.

leukemia, the gallium scan is useful in detecting extramedullary sites of tumor involvement. Gallium does not localize in involved nodes in chronic lymphocytic leukemia. These findings fit well with the concept that gallium localizes in tissue by binding to lactoferrin (see Chapter 1). Granulocytes are rich in lactoferrin, whereas lymphocytes contain little or none of this protein.

REFERENCES

1.   Luce JK, McBride CM, Frei E III: Melanoma, in Cancer Medicine, Holland JL, Frei E III (eds), Philadelphia, Lea and Febiger, 1973, pp. 1832–1843.

2.   Milder MS, Frankel RS, Gregory B, et al: Gallium-67 scintigraphy in malignant melanoma. *Cancer* **32**:1350, 1973.

3.   Jackson FI, McPherson A, Lentle BC: Gallium-67 scintigraphy in multisystem malignant melanoma. *Radiology* **122**:163, 1977.

4.   Jewel KL: Primary carcinoma of the liver, clinical and radiologic manifestations. *Amer J Roentgenol Radium Ther Nucl Med* **113**:84, 1971.

5.   Suzuki T, Honjo I, Hamamoto K, et al: Positive scintiphotography of cancer of the liver with ^{67}Ga citrate. *Amer J Roentgenol Radium Ther Nucl Med* **113**:92, 1971.

6.   Lomas F, Dibos PE, Wagner HN Jr: Increased specificity of liver scanning with the use of gallium-67 citrate. *N Engl J Med* **286**:1323, 1972.

7.   Hamamoto K, Torizuka K, Mukai T, et al: Usefulness of computer scintigraphy for detecting liver tumor with ^{67}Ga citrate and the scintillation camera. *J Nucl Med* **13**:667, 1972.

8.   Suzuki T, Matsumoto Y, Manabe T, et al: Serum α-fetoprotein and ^{67}Ga-citrate uptake in hepatoma. *Amer J Roentgenol Radium Ther Nucl Med* **120**:627, 1974.

9.   Levin J, Kew MC: Gallium-67 citrate scanning in primary cancer of the liver: diagnostic value in the presence of cirrhosis and relation to alpha-fetoprotein. *J Nucl Med* **16**:949, 1975.

10. Hammersley PAG, Zivanovic MA: Gallium-67 uptake in the regenerating rat liver. *J Nucl Med* **17**:226, 1976.

11. Hill JH, Wagner HN: ^{67}Ga-uptake in the regenerating rat liver. *J Nucl Med* **15**:818, 1974.

12. Hammersley PAG, Cauch MN, Taylor DM: Gallium uptake in the regenerating rat liver and its relationship to lysosomal enzyme activity. *Cancer Res* **35**:1154, 1975.

13. Belanger MA, Beauchamp JM, Neiteschman HR: Gallium uptake in benign tumor of liver: case report. *J Nucl Med* **16**:470, 1975.

14. Chauncey DM, Halpern SE, Hagan PL, et al: Tumor model studies of ^{131}tetracyline and other compounds. *J Nucl Med* **17**:274, 1976.

15. Gelrud LG, Arseneau JC, Milder MS, et al: The kinetics of ^{67}Ga incorporation into inflammatory lesions: experimental and clinical studies. *J Lab Clin Med* **83**:489, 1974.

16. Arseneau JC, Aamodt R, Johnston GS, et al: Evidence for granulocytic incorporation of ^{67}Ga in chronic granulocytic leukemia. *J Lab Clin Med* **83**:495, 1974.

12

Organ Systems in Which Gallium-67 Is of Limited Utility

Paul B. Hoffer, M.D.

Professor of Diagnostic Radiology
Director, Section of Nuclear Medicine
Yale University School of Medicine
New Haven, Connecticut

Steven M. Pinsky, M.D.

Director, Division of Nuclear Medicine
Michael Reese Hospital and Medical Center

Associate Professor of Radiology
University of Chicago
Pritzker School of Medicine

Chicago, Illinois

The organ systems discussed in this chapter are those in which gallium scanning plays only a minor role in tumor detection and staging. In some cases, gallium is taken up by the lesion, but other more sensitive and specific detection or staging procedures are available. In most cases, gallium has only limited affinity for the tumor tissue itself.

THYROID

Only about 25% of solitary "cold" nodules detected on conventional radioiodine or ^{99m}Tc pertechnetate thyroid scans are malignant. A simple technique to differentiate the benign from the malignant cold nodules would eliminate the need for surgery in most patients with benign nodules.

The early reports of Langhammer et al. (1) suggested that gallium-67 (^{67}Ga) might be helpful in the diagnosis of thyroid cancer. Seven of eight patients in their series with thyroid carcinoma had positive gallium scans; six of the seven were verified surgically. The five patients who had received no prior treatment of thyroid carcinoma all had positive gallium accumulation; the group included two patients with anaplastic carcinoma of the thyroid. There are now 10 studies in which a total of 63 patients with thyroid cancer have been evaluated by ^{67}Ga scans (Table 1). Only 27 of these 63, or about 40%, had positive gallium scans. An unusually high proportion of the positive scans in these series occurred in patients with anaplastic carcinoma of the thyroid. In the series reported by Kaplan et al. (2), two of the three positive scans were anaplastic carcinomas; the other carcinoma was a mixed papillary-follicular type. In the series reported by Erjavec et al. (3), all three positive scans were in patients with anaplastic carcinomas. Three of four of the scans in patients with papillary or follicular carcinomas were negative, and the other showed only minimal uptake of gallium. In Koutras et al.'s study (4), one of the two malignancies that accumulated gallium

TABLE 1   POSITIVE THYROID SCANS IN PATIENTS WITH MALIGNANT
THYROID LESIONS

Series	Year	Malignant Thyroid Scans	Number Detected
Edwards and Hayes (19)	1970	2	0
Berelowitz and Blake (20)	1971	1	0
Higasi et al. (15)	1972	4	1
Langhammer et al. (1)	1972	8	7
Roos and Shoot (7)	1973	5	3
Manfredi et al. (5)	1973	5	3
Kaplan et al. (2)	1974	7	3
Erjavec et al. (3)	1974	7	3
Heifdendal et al. (21)	1975	16	5
Koutras et al. (4)	1976	8	2
Total		63	27

was an anaplastic carcinoma. All three of the carcinomas that accumulated gallium in the Manfred et al. series (5) were also anaplastic. Anaplastic carcinoma is one of the more rare histologic types of malignant thyroid tumor. The proportion of anaplastic carcinomas in the reported series of patients studied with ^{67}Ga is quite high. Therefore, the overall detectability of thyroid tumors by gallium scan is probably even lower than the 35–45% value suggested in the literature.

Gallium is only rarely taken up in benign thyroid nodules. Only five of a group of 113 surgically proven benign nodules took up gallium. In three of these five cases, the uptake was only slight. Gallium is, however, taken up avidly by inflammatory thyroid lesions, including thyroiditis (6).

Erjavec and associates (3) have quantitatively determined ^{67}Ga uptake in normal and abnormal thyroid tissue. They have observed that the normal thyroid tissue to background ratio of ^{67}Ga is about 2:1 (see Table 2). The only diseases that demonstrated significant deviations from this were anaplastic carcinoma (5:1) and thyroiditis (3:1).

Roos and Shoot (7) have studied gallium uptake in euthyroid patients with multinodular goiter. Of 13 patients examined, five were shown at surgery to have carcinoma. Three of these patients had positive gallium scans. In addition, two patients with metastatic thyroid disease had gallium scans that were positive in skull metastases, and one patient with leiomyosarcoma of the thyroid had abnormal uptake of ^{67}Ga in the lesion.

While routine gallium scan does not appear indicated for differentiation of cold nodules of the thyroid, it may be of value in certain specific situations. A positive scan is strongly suggestive of malignancy, but a negative scan does not indicate that the lesion is benign. The avidity of ^{67}Ga for thyroid tissue involved

TABLE 2   UPTAKE OF GALLIUM CITRATE IN NECK STRUCTURES:
45 OBSERVATIONS IN 22 PATIENTS*

Structures	Number of Observations	Structure to Neck Background Ratio[†]	
		Mean	Range
Normal thyroid tissue	7	2.1	1.5-2.3
Suppressed thyroid tissue	2	1.7	1.7
Manubrium sterni	14	1.7	1.6-2.0
Autonomous/toxic adenoma	2	1.75	1.7-1.8
Thyroiditis chronica	4	3.1	1.3-5.2
Nodular goiter with regressive changes	9	1.4	1.0-1.8
Lymphadenitis tuberculosa	1	2.2	
Papillary-follicular carcinoma	4	1.7	1.2-2.3
Medullary carcinoma	1	2.0	
Anaplastic carcinoma	1	4.7	
Total	45		

*From Erjavec et al. (3).
[†]The structure to neck background ratios were determined by means of computer-processed images.

with thyroiditis may be helpful in distinguishing between that diagnosis and hemorrhage in a patient who presents with a painful thyroid nodule.

OTHER HEAD AND NECK LESIONS

Silberstein and associates (8) studied a group of patients with squamous cell tumors of the head and neck to determine if gallium scanning was useful for detection or staging of their disease. Only 15 of 22 unirradiated tumors were detectable by scan. All of the lesions detectable by scan were also observable by other diagnostic methods. They concluded that gallium was not useful in evaluating nonlymphomatous head and neck lesions prior to treatment. Their study also included 12 patients with residual tumor following preoperative irradiation. Three of the patients' scans demonstrated uptake of gallium in the recurrent lesion. All three patients died within 6 months of the scan, whereas the nine patients without gallium uptake in the residual tumor were all alive 8–14 months after treatment.

Higasi and coworkers (9) have observed that the gallium scan is useful in differentiating maxillary carcinoma from chronic sinusitis. All 14 cases of squamous cell carcinoma, in addition to three of four other maxillary sinus tumors, were strongly positive on gallium scan. Seven patients with chronic sinusitis and no tumor had negative or only weakly positive gallium scans. These findings are surprising, because gallium is usually taken up avidly in areas of inflammation.

BRAIN

Gallium imaging has been investigated for use in detection and evaluation of both primary and metastatic brain tumors (5,10,11,12). Manfredi and associates (5) report detection of 14 of 15 primary brain tumors and nine of 11 metastatic lesions. Jones and colleagues identified 15 of 17 primary brain tumors in their first reported series (10) and four of five primary tumors in their second series (11). Despite these excellent results, the gallium scan is not superior to the conventional ^{99m}Tc pertechnetate scan for detection of primary tumors. No direct comparisons with computed tomography imaging have been performed. Since gallium uptake in brain lesions is also nonspecific (see Chapter 6), it provides no information that is not obtainable with the current methods used for detection of primary brain tumors.

Gallium may, however, be useful in the evaluation of metastatic tumors and in the postoperative evaluation of primary brain tumors. Metastatic skull lesions are not well delineated on ^{99m}Tc pertechnetate images obtained 1–2 hours after injection of the radionuclide. These lesions are easily observable on gallium scans. Therefore, the gallium scan will detect calvarial metastatic lesions missed by conventional brain scans.

Paradoxically, gallium scanning is useful in the postoperative evaluation of brain tumors because it is not taken up in the periphery of the craniotomy defect as avidly is as ^{99m}Tc pertechnetate. The gallium scan provides a truer picture of the extent of the residual or recurrent lesion than does the ^{99m}Tc pertechnetate image.

GASTROINTESTINAL TRACT

Gallium is not useful for the detection or staging of gastrointestinal tract tumors. Langhammer and associates (1) reported uptake of gallium in only 14 of 33 tumors. Silberstein's review of the literature in 1976 (3) revealed only 30 of 78 cases of gallium-positive gastrointestinal tumors. This review also revealed only two of 14 pancreatic tumors and only seven of 17 eosophageal tumors that were positive on gallium scan. The low incidence of positive gallium scans in gastrointestinal tumors is surprising, because both the small bowel and the colon actually secrete gallium. It is possible that the poor results may be due to an inability to distinguish normal gut activity from tumor uptake. It is interesting that the poor results with gallium scanning in the intestinal tract occur with both adenocarcinomas and squamous cell lesions (3).

BREAST

Gallium is taken up in the breasts of lactating women, presumably because of its binding to lactoferrin, a milk protein. Gallium scanning has been investigated as a method of detection and staging of breast cancer (1,13,–17). A summary of the detection rates as reported in the literature is presented in Table 3. Only about 50% of primary breast tumors are detectable on the ^{67}Ga scan. Also, ^{67}Ga is occasionally taken up in the breast tissue of women who do not have malignant breast tumors and who are not lactating (17,18). Therefore, gallium has not proven useful as a method for early detection of carcinoma of the breast.

Richman and associates at the National Institutes of Health (16) have also evaluated gallium scanning as a method of staging breast cancer. The gallium scan detected metastatic lesions in only 54 of 83 (65%) patients with known metastatic tumor. It was less sensitive than the liver scan (8% versus 80%) in detecting liver metastasis, less sensitive than the bone scan and radiography (65% versus 100%) for detection of bone metastasis, less sensitive than the brain scan (20% versus 40%) for detection of brain metastasis, and less sensitive than the chest x-ray (35% versus 100%) for detection of pulmonary metastasis. The gallium scan was useful, however, in detecting mediastinal spread of tumor. Eight of nine patients with mediastinal tumor were detected on scan. X-ray and mediastinal tomography were normal in three of the eight patients with positive scans. Based on these results, Richman and associates feel that gallium is useful in staging patients with breast cancer.

TABLE 3   UPTAKE OF GALLIUM IN PRIMARY BREAST TUMORS

Series	Total Number of Cases	Positive	Equivocal	Negative
Lavender et al. (14)	4	0	—	4
Higasi et al. (15)	16	8	2	6
Richman et al. (16)	21	11	—	10
Richman et al. (17)	10	5	—	5

GENITOURINARY TRACT

Except for its use in staging testicular tumors (see chapter 9), evaluation of gallium for detection of genitourinary tract lesions has been limited and disappointing. Langhammer et al. reported that only three of 13 genitourinary tumors had positive uptake on gallium scan (1).

CONCLUSION

It is difficult to explain why some tumors take up gallium and others do not. Inflammatory response to the tumor may play some role but does not provide a total answer. Hopefully, future studies of tumor metabolism, including evaluation of the role of metal-binding proteins, will help us to understand why gallium goes where it does and also aid in the design of new and better agents for tumor detection.

REFERENCES

1. Langhammer H, Glaubitt G, Grebe SF, et al: ^{67}Ga for tumor scanning. *J Nucl Med* **13**:25, 1972.

2. Kaplan WD, Holman BL, Selenkow HA, et al: ^{67}Ga citrate and the non-functioning thyroid nodule. *J Nucl Med* **15**:424, 1974

3. Erjavec M, Auersperg M, Golouh R, et al: Computer assisted scanning in evaluation of ^{67}Ga citrate in thyroid disease. *J Nucl Med* **15**:810, 1974.

4. Koutras DA, Pandos PG, Stontouris J: Thyroid scanning with gallium-67 and cesium 131. *J Nucl Med* **17**:268, 1976.

5. Manfredi OL, Quiones JD, Bartok SP: Tumor detection with gallium-67 citrate, in Medical Radioisotope Scintigraphy, Vol 2, Vienna, International Atomic Energy Agency (IAEA-SM-164/208), 1973, p. 583.

6. Grove RB, Pinsky SM, Brown TL, et al: Uptake of ^{67}Ga-citrate in subacute thyroiditis. *J Nucl Med* **14**:403, 1973.

7. Roos J, Shoot JB: The uptake of gallium-67 in euthyroid patients with multinodular goiter. *Acta Med Scand* **194**:225, 1973.

8. Silberstein EG, Kornblut A, Shumrich K, et al: ^{67}Ga as a diagnostic agent for the detection of head and neck tumors and lymphoma. *Radiology* **110**:605, 1974.

9. Higasi T, Auyama W, Mori Y, et al: Gallium-67 scanning in the differentiation of maxillary sinus carcinoma from chronic maxillary sinusitis. *Radiology* **123**:117, 1977.

10. Jones AE, Koslow M, Johnston GS, et al: ^{67}Ga citrate scintigraphy of brain tumors. *Radiology* **105**:693, 1972.

11. Jones EA, Frankel RS, Di Chiro G, et al: Brain Scintigraphy with ^{99m}Tc-pertechnetate, ^{99m}Tc-polyphosphate and ^{67}Ga citrate. *Radiology* **112**:123, 1974.

12. Henkin RE, Quinn JL, Weinberg PE: Adjunctive brain scanning with ^{67}Ga in metastases. *Radiology* **106**:595, 1973.

13. Silberstein EB: Cancer diagnosis: the role of tumor imaging radiopharmaceuticals. *Amer J Med* **60**:226, 1974.

14. Lavender JP, Lowe J, Barker JR, et al: Gallium-67 citrate scanning in neoplastic and inflammatory lesions. *Brit J Radiol* **44**:361, 1971.

15. Higasi T, Nakayama Y, Murata A, et al: Clinical Evaluation of ^{67}Ga citrate scanning. *J Nucl Med* **13**:196, 1972.

16. Richman SD, Ingle XX, Levenson XX, et al: Usefulness of gallium scintigraphy in primary and metastatic breast cancer. *J Nucl Med* **16**:996, 1975.

17. Richman SD, Brodey PA, Frankel RS, et al: Breast scintigraphy with ^{99m}Tc-pertechnetate and ^{67}Ga-citrate. *J Nucl Med* **16**:293, 1076.

18. Hor G, Heidenreich P, Kriegel XX, et al: Breast scintigraphy with 99mTc-pertechnetate and 67Ga-citrate (Letters to the editor). *J. Nucl Med* **17**:223, 1976.

19. Edwards CL, Hayes RL: Scanning malignant neoplasms with gallium-67. *J Amer Med Assn* **212**:1182, 1970.

20. Berelowitz M, Blake KCH: 67Gallium in the detection and localization of tumors. *S Afr Med J* **45**:1351, 1971.

21. Heidendal GAK, Roos P, Thijs LG, et al: Evaluation of cold areas on the thyroid scan with 67Ga-citrate. *J Nucl Med* **16**:793, 1975.

Index

Proceedings of The British Institute of Radiology

Thirty-eighth Annual Congress, April 17–18, 1980

Isotopes in oncology

The following abstract was inadvertently omitted from the Proceedings published in The British Journal of Radiology, 53 1114–16 (November 1980). We apologize for any inconvenience caused.

TUMOUR LOCALIZATION WITH GALLIUM-67 AND INDIUM-111 RADIOPHARMACEUTICALS

By D. M. Taylor

University of Heidelberg and Kernforschungszentrum Karlsruhe, Institut für Genetik und für Toxikologie von Spaltstoffen, Postfach 3640 D 7500 Karlsruhe 1, Federal Republic of Germany

^{67}Ga citrate and ^{111}In-Bleomycin have been in clinical use for more than a decade. Neither of these radiopharmaceuticals are tumour-specific and uptake occurs in all normal tissues and in many sites of infection.

Both agents concentrate to some extent in a wide range of tumours, but the uptake may be quite variable in tumours of the same histological class, both between different patients and between different tumour sites within the same patient. In general ^{111}In-Bleomycin is no better, or is inferior to ^{67}Ga citrate for tumour visualization, except perhaps for the tent ^{111}In, are useful in establishing a differential diagnosis, particularly in the chest and in the differentiation between seminoma and teratoma. ^{67}Ga is also useful in delineating the total extent of malignant disease especially around the mediastinum, where neither X rays nor CAT scans provide good information, and in the staging of Hodgkin's disease and the lymphomas.

They cannot however provide a primary diagnostic screen. The physiological mechanisms underlying the uptake of gallium and indium by tumours are still incompletely understood. Their uptake appears to be directly related to lysosomal enzyme activity in tumours and normal tissues and other important factors are plasma and lysosomal membrane permeability and transferrin.

Rapidly growing tissues tend to show both increased cell permeability and lysosomal activity compared to slowly growing or resting tissues. Thus a "^{67}Ga-avid tumour" is probably more "active" than a tumour showing only weak ^{67}Ga uptake. Radiation or chemotherapy which retards or inhibits tumour growth also reduces ^{67}Ga uptake. This reduction of loss of ^{67}Ga concentrating ability by a tumour, measured by serial quantitative scans, may provide a useful index of the response of the tumour to treatment and of prognosis.

Since the accumulation of ^{67}Ga citrate or ^{111}In-Bleomycin by a tumour is a dynamic process, these two expensive radiopharmaceuticals can be exploited to yield useful functional information about the tumour, in addition to a static image of the tumour distribution, and this should be the major objective of future studies with these two radionuclides.